HOW TO EAT TO BEAT DISEASE COOKBOOK

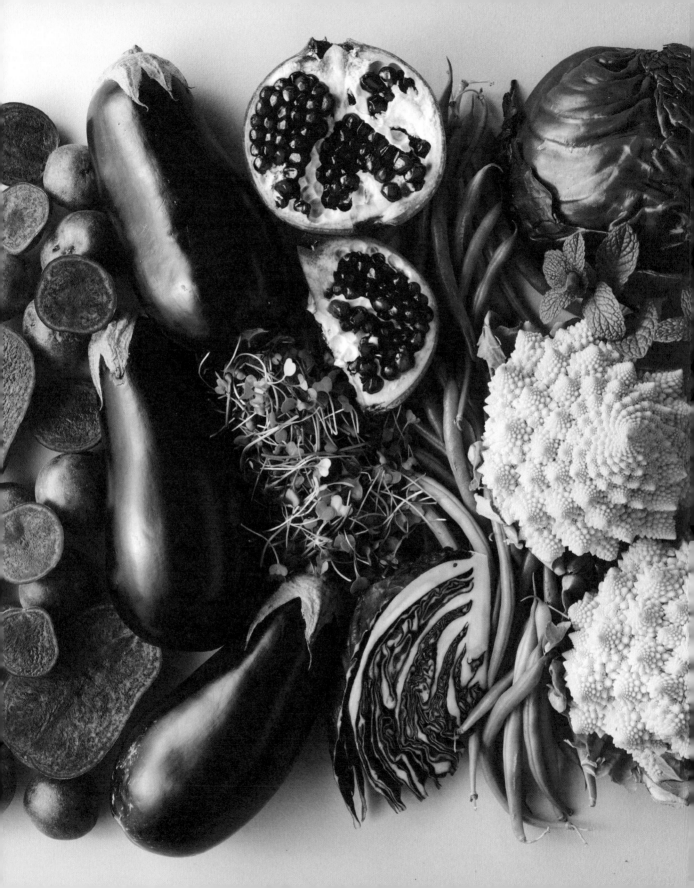

HOW TO
EAT to BEAT DISEASE
COOKBOOK

75 Healthy Recipes to Protect Your Well-Being
INCLUDES A 14-DAY MEAL PLAN

Ginger Hultin, MS, RDN

Photography by Marija Vidal

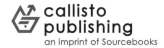
callisto
publishing
an imprint of Sourcebooks

Copyright © 2021 by Callisto Publishing LLC

Cover and internal design © 2021 by Callisto Publishing LLC

Photography © 2021 Marija Vidal. Food styling by Elisabet der Nederlanden.

Interior and Cover Designer: Stephanie Sumulong and Emma Hall

Art Producer: Sue Bischofberger

Editor: Rebecca Markley

Published by Callisto Publishing LLC C/O Sourcebooks LLC

P.O. Box 4410, Naperville, Illinois 60567-4410

(630) 961-3900

callistopublishing.com

Printed and Bound In China

OGP 16

To my Mom, Cheryle, and Gram and
and Grandpa Weiss, who have always
known that food heals and who have
inspired me to do this work.

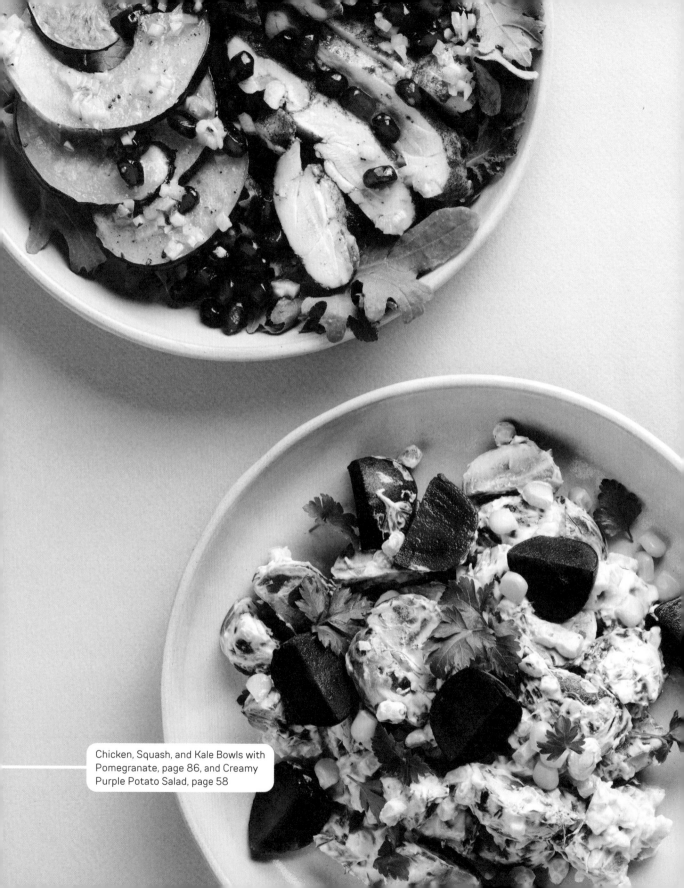

Chicken, Squash, and Kale Bowls with Pomegranate, page 86, and Creamy Purple Potato Salad, page 58

CONTENTS

INTRODUCTION

The body has powerful systems in place to keep us healthy and prevent disease. As a registered dietitian nutritionist, I've committed my life to helping people use food and other lifestyle factors to optimize their body's natural mechanisms. My master's degree in nutrition is from Bastyr University in the Seattle area, whose program puts a special emphasis on how food can help heal the body. This foundation of an integrative, holistic approach to health combined with years of clinical practice has fueled my interest in how food affects the body.

There has been a lot of research done on the impact of food on specific diseases. It has revealed that individual foods offer promise, while overall eating patterns offer insight into what may be best for human health. For example, large, long-term, human studies have shown that vegetarian and vegan diets can reduce the risk of ischemic heart disease, type 2 diabetes, high blood pressure, obesity, and even certain types of cancer (Melina, Craig, and Levin 2016). The Dietary Approaches to Stop Hypertension (DASH) diet has also repeatedly been shown, in large clinical trials, to effectively lower blood pressure as well as the risk of cardiac events (like heart attacks), strokes, type 2 diabetes, and obesity (Challa, Ameer, and Uppaluri 2018). The Mediterranean diet has been found to reduce cardiovascular disease, type 2 diabetes, brain functioning issues and cognitive decline, depression, and several types of cancer (Sánchez-Sánchez et al. 2020). What do all of these diets have in common? They're based on whole, unprocessed foods, and they emphasize high-fiber options including fruits and vegetables. The Mediterranean and DASH diets include plant proteins as well as some lean animal protein like chicken and fish. All of the diets are low in saturated fat, added salt, and added sugar.

These dietary themes support the same principles that Dr. William Li presents in his best-selling book *Eat to Beat Disease: The New Science of How Your Body Can Heal Itself*. Using some of his own research on angiogenesis and cancer-fighting foods, he provides a comprehensive analysis of a wide range of studies that show how diet can be used to bolster our natural defense systems. Taking a holistic approach, he does a deep dive into exactly what foods to eat—and to avoid—for optimal health. His focus is on supporting the body's existing healing systems through diet and lifestyle. As a registered dietitian nutritionist, I take the same approach.

The purpose behind this cookbook is to provide you with easy and delicious ways to include more foods that support your health every day. Although it is important that you choose foods mindfully, this eating plan is not meant to be strict or restrictive. I encourage you to move away from the mindset of cutting foods out of your diet and focus instead on adding foods. After all, food is part of the fun and joy of life.

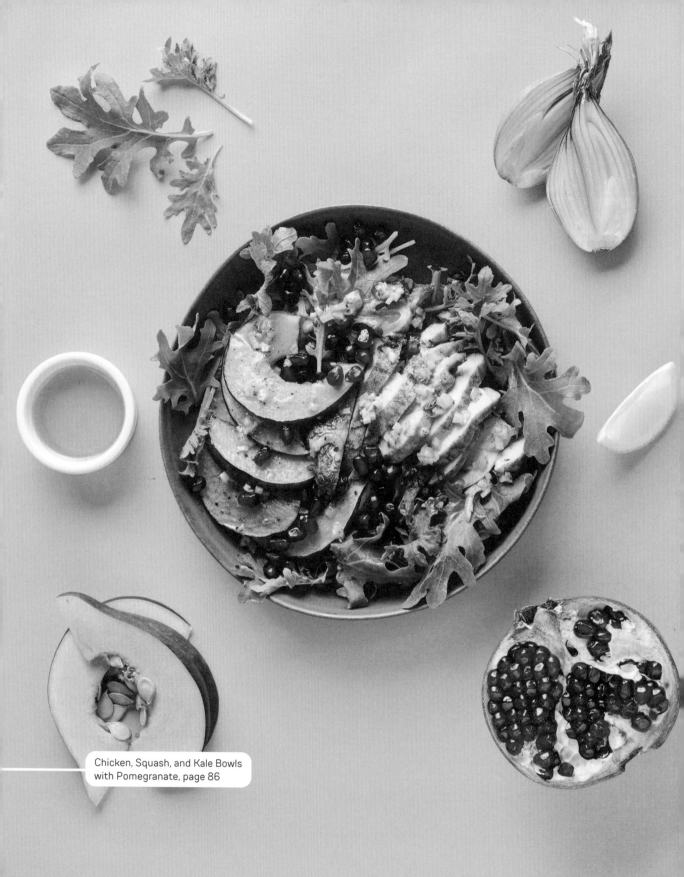

Chicken, Squash, and Kale Bowls with Pomegranate, page 86

How to Use This Book

This book is organized to help you navigate how to eat to beat disease, with specific meal plan guidance and recipes that include foods in the different categories that help boost the body's natural defenses against disease.

Chapter 1 reviews the five major defense systems in the body, including how they work and how they can go wrong. It also offers a synopsis of how food can support each of the five systems to promote optimal health. The information presented is an overview of current research and the ways we can help the body heal itself and prevent disease. For a deeper exploration into each system and to better understand the breadth of research on each subject, please refer to Dr. Li's book *Eat to Beat Disease*.

Chapter 2 includes a comprehensive food list and strategies for incorporating these foods into your own life. You can use the list to quickly identify which foods fall into which category of disease prevention. The chapter also includes a 14-day meal plan and shopping lists to help you get off to a smooth start.

Chapters 3 through 8 include 75 recipes that are specifically designed to support your health, including recipes for breakfasts, main meals, and even sweet treats. As you review the recipes, feel free to swap in foods from the food list in Chapter 2 for variety or to accommodate your likes and dislikes or food allergies. You can also add more foods from the list for increased health benefits. The *How to Eat to Beat Disease Cookbook* is designed to be versatile and support a wide variety of dietary preferences.

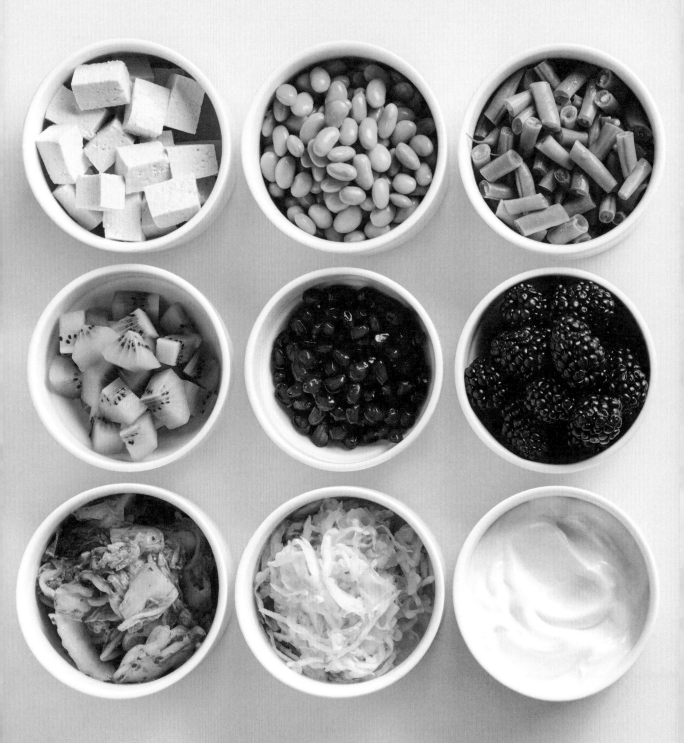

CHAPTER 1

The Body's Defense Systems Against Disease

Dr. Li presents the concept of health as an active state protected by the complex interaction of the five major defense systems: angiogenesis, cell regeneration, microbiome health, DNA protection, and the immune system. In his book, he presents an in-depth analysis of research on each of these topics. As with all bodily systems, these defense systems work synergistically.

For the purposes of this book, I'll provide an overview of each system, explain what happens when one is not working correctly, and highlight the foods that provide the greatest benefits within each system.

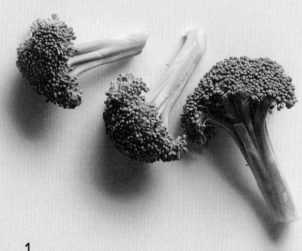

Angiogenesis

Simply put, angiogenesis is the process of blood vessel formation. Angiogenesis is important because the body has a natural ability to regulate when and where new blood vessels are produced in order to increase or decrease the blood supply to various parts of the body as needed. This system plays a critical role in maintaining healthy tissue, healing damaged tissue, and preventing the growth and spread of potential cancer cells.

WHEN ANGIOGENESIS IS COMPROMISED

Disease can result from excessive angiogenesis, which is when blood vessels feed diseased tissue or cancerous tumors, and insufficient angiogenesis, which is when there aren't enough blood vessels to supply healthy tissue with the blood and nutrients it needs to survive.

Excessive angiogenesis can lead to blindness from age-related macular degeneration and diabetes-related vision loss (Penn et al. 2008). There is also evidence that too much angiogenesis can lead to the worsening of rheumatoid arthritis, an autoimmune disease that causes inflammation in the joints (Bousseau et al. 2018). Medications that inhibit excessive angiogenesis are now a common type of cancer therapy (Saeed et al. 2019).

Diabetes is a disease that can cause insufficient angiogenesis, which can reduce the blood supply to nerves when blood sugar is not properly controlled. Lack of angiogenesis can also cause chronic wounds and subsequent infections because inadequate blood flow to the affected area impedes healing (Okonkwo and DiPietro 2017).

Well-balanced angiogenesis is essential for preserving health and preventing disease. It is necessary for getting proper blood supply to organs like your brain and heart, even helping the body naturally work around blockages through new blood vessel formation (Potz et al. 2017). It is equally important in cutting off the fuel supply that cancer cells need for rapid growth.

BALANCING ANGIOGENESIS THROUGH FOOD

Luckily, the foods we eat can help prevent or slow chronic diseases that are caused by both excessive and insufficient angiogenesis. Many foods can help the body regulate this defense system to optimize proper blood flow while stopping blood vessels from forming abnormally to feed diseased tissue or cause other damage. Whether you're eating angiogenic (blood vessel–forming) or antiangiogenic (blood vessel–regulating) foods, you'll improve your overall health. Specific foods that can help the body manage angiogenesis include soy, tomatoes, green tea, kale, and pomegranates, among many others that you can find on Your Eat to Beat Disease Food List (page 17).

Soy?! Yes, Soy

Some people may be surprised to see soy foods recommended so strongly in Dr. Li's book and throughout this cookbook as well. There is so much misinformation and fear around this food, and it's time to clear it up.

Soy foods are a staple in diets around the world, but especially in China, Singapore, and Japan. This has allowed large, long-term, human studies on the health risks and benefits of consuming them.

Soy foods (and many other foods we eat) contain antioxidants called isoflavones, which are *phytoestrogens*, or plant estrogens. Though not exactly the same as human and animal estrogens, they are similar in structure and actually work as estrogen modulators. They have shown anticancer support in addition to health benefits for the heart and bones. The American Cancer Society and other major cancer organizations have statements about the safety of soy, so it really is time to change our tune about this incredibly healthy food.

Cell Regeneration

Cells in all tissue and organs are constantly being maintained and repaired, and the body must be able to regenerate cells as needed in order to survive. Whereas angiogenesis is the process of growing new blood vessels to support healthy tissue, stem cells are the way that the intestines, lungs, skin, blood cells, and even your bones are renewed throughout your life. Cells in the colon regenerate every four days, which is relatively quick. Some white blood cells live for about a year (others have a much shorter lifespan), whereas red blood cells survive for about three months, and platelets only last for about 12 days. The body's natural ability to regenerate cells is a key to survival, and certain foods contain compounds that can help support the process.

THE SPECIAL POWERS OF STEM CELLS

Stem cells are the engine that powers regeneration in the body. Stem cells in adults are not specialized but remain ready to regenerate when needed due to injury or illness in organs and tissue in the body. Many stem cells are stored in the bone marrow and are activated by an enzyme called vascular endothelial growth factor (VEGF). Stem cells are guided to the place they're needed through cell-to-cell communication. Once they arrive at their destination, they transform into the heart, skin, or other organ tissue they were called to regenerate.

One example of how amazing stem cells are is one that you may already be familiar with: a stem cell transplant for a person going through cancer treatment, which is a lifesaving therapy. It is done by transferring stem cells from a donor to a patient with cancer in the hope that the donor's stem cells will help the patient's body make healthy new blood cells. Cure rates of some blood cancers are now around 90%, thanks to stem cell therapy.

Stem cells also support your heart and vascular system. If there's a blockage or the blood flow through arteries or into the heart is compromised, vascular stem cells help regenerate blood vessels to get critical nutrients and oxygen to the right tissues.

Stem cells can be damaged by chronic diseases, such as type 2 diabetes, or by lifestyle factors like smoking tobacco and excessive alcohol intake. This damage can lead to regeneration dysfunction, but the good news is that there are many foods you can eat that support healthy stem cells.

SUPPORTING CELL REGENERATION THROUGH FOOD

Cocoa powder, which is rich in antioxidants, supports healthy stem cell recruitment. Anti-inflammatory omega-3 fatty acids, found in some fish as well as plant foods like flaxseed, chia, hempseed, and walnuts, have been shown in studies to help stem cells function better by migrating around the body with more ease. In *Eat to Beat Disease*, Dr. Li analyzes research on how other foods, including whole wheat, green beans, rice bran, and turmeric, support stem cells and regeneration in the body. In addition, foods that are high in certain antioxidants like resveratrol (red wine!), zeaxanthin (corn, kale, mustard greens, and other leafy vegetables), and chlorogenic acid (coffee, black tea, and blueberries) have been shown in studies to help stem cells regenerate tissues in the body.

Several types of beverages can help stem cells circulate in the body more efficiently, and two of them contain alcohol: red wine and beer. This could possibly be because alcohol slightly thins the blood, and these beverages also contain a lot of unique antioxidants. If you abstain from alcohol, you still have options. Both green and black tea have been found to boost the number of stem cells circulating in the body (Fujiki et al. 2018; Mitra and Khandelwal 2017).

Microbiome Health

You've got a very large community of bacteria—in the trillions—residing in your intestines. This is called the gut microbiome. Research continues to explore how these bacteria support human health (Mohajeri et al. 2018). The interaction between the gut microbiome and health is complex. For example, the types of bacteria you have in your colon change through life stages, pregnancy, diet changes, and medications you take, especially antibiotics. Gut bacteria create metabolites (substances) that actually affect brain signaling and the immune system. By feeding the gut micro-biome with healthy prebiotics and probiotics, you can keep this system working optimally, which is a key factor in protecting your health.

WHEN GUT HEALTH GOES WRONG

There are a lot of potential threats to the health of your gut micro-biome, including certain diseases in the digestive tract, a diet that doesn't properly feed the bacteria living there, and some medications. When gut bacteria become altered, serious diseases, including inflamma-tory bowel diseases, such as Crohn's disease and ulcerative colitis, can develop. Alterations in gut bacteria can also affect the cardiovascular and immune systems.

Food allergies can also cause problems with the gut. For example, although high-fiber whole wheat would normally help the body's natural defense systems, for those with celiac disease, it can damage health. When the immune system identifies gluten (the protein found in wheat) as a threat, a person with celiac disease will have an immune reaction in the gut that causes diarrhea or constipation (or both), weight loss, bloating, gas, and abdominal pain when they eat wheat.

SUPPORTING MICROBIOME HEALTH THROUGH FOOD

Although there's a lot still to be learned about the microbiome, like which bacteria are potentially beneficial and harmful, what ratios are optimal, and which individual strains may be ideal for human health, research does point to the fact that diversity in the bacteria seems to be positive. To foster diversity and keep the bacteria "happy," it's important to include foods that naturally contain microbes. This includes eating foods with pro-biotics, such as fermented foods, as well as foods with prebiotic fiber that support gut bacteria, like fruits, vegetables, whole grains, and beans.

Many culinary traditions around the world include foods that are prepared by bacterial fermentation, and there's evidence that this process is beneficial to the gut, providing a dietary source of live microorganisms that may support the microbiome defense system. Kimchi, sauerkraut, and pao cai (Sichuan fermented pickle, usually made from cabbage) contain potentially beneficial microbes, in addition to being high-fiber foods (Marco et al. 2017). Cheese is also made using a starter culture that utilizes different bacterial strains. There's some evidence that cheese, like Parmigiano-Reggiano, Gouda, and Camembert, can positively affect the bacterial biodiversity of those who consume it (Milani et al. 2019). Other fermented dairy products, like yogurt and kefir, have been shown to influence the gut microbiome within a month of consuming them daily (Volokh et al. 2019). Even sourdough bread, made with a bacterial starter (*Lactobacillus*), which is ultimately cooked and does not contain live bacteria, could be helpful to human health by supporting the immune system (Zheng et al. 2015).

DNA Health

Your genetic blueprint is unique just to you. It is kept inside DNA in every cell in your body and is important to protect from damage. DNA is made of genes inherited from your parents that defend your body by telling it how to function optimally throughout your life. There are a lot of threats to your DNA health, including chemical and environmental exposure and even lack of sleep or exercise, that can lead to DNA damage and a weakening of this powerful defense system.

THREATS TO DNA HEALTH

DNA damage can happen at high levels with normal exposures during daily life. For example, ultraviolet (UV) rays from the sun can do a lot of damage, increasing your risk of skin cancer. Smoking tobacco—either first- or second-hand exposure—is damaging to DNA because of compounds such as polycyclic aromatic hydrocarbons (PAHs) and nitrosamines, which can lead to increased risk of cancers of the mouth, throat, esophagus, stomach, colon, rectum, liver, pancreas, larynx, trachea, bronchus, kidney, bladder, cervix, and more.

PAHs and another toxic compound, heterocyclic amines (HCAs), are a common exposure that damages DNA when charred beef, pork, fish, and poultry are consumed. PAHs are also found in smoked foods.

Part of DNA protection has to do with the ends of chromosomes (the structures made of DNA found in the nucleus of every cell), telomeres, which are the protective caps on the ends of DNA strands. There is important research on what can harm telomeres, damaging DNA and leading to an increased risk of certain cancers, and what can protect them. A lot of that has to do with diet. Studies on soda consumption in children have shown that it shortens telomeres (Wojcicki et al. 2018), whereas studies on the intake of antioxidant-rich foods and omega-3 fatty acids have shown that they offer protection (Prasad, Wu, and Bondy 2017).

SUPPORTING DNA HEALTH THROUGH FOOD

The most important foods that help protect against DNA damage fall into three categories: those high in antioxidants that help protect DNA, those with epigenetic effects that may help repair broken DNA or influence DNA function, and those that help protect telomeres.

Research has identified that juices from fruits like grapes, pomegranates, cherries, and blackberries can protect against DNA damage, as can kiwi, carrots, broccoli, and foods rich in the compound lycopene (tomatoes, watermelons, guava, pink grapefruit).

Foods rich in omega-3 fatty acids, including salmon, hake, sea cucumber, manila clams, tuna, yellowtail, walnuts, chia, hemp, and flaxseed, have anti-inflammatory effects and help improve DNA repair in cells.

Still other foods contain compounds that actually influence how DNA functions by activating and deactivating it as needed. Foods with this unique ability include soy, cruciferous vegetables (broccoli, cauliflower, Brussels sprouts, kale, cabbage, etc.), coffee, green tea, turmeric, and herbs like basil, marjoram, sage, thyme, and peppermint.

Immune System

One of the body's most important defenses is a robust immune system, which plays a protective role in fighting off disease. Because of the complex nature of how this system works, there are many factors that could negatively affect it. Immunodeficiency diseases (there are more than 300) are caused by defects in the immune system and can cause recurrent infections. Though rare, they still affect 1 in 100,000 people, not including those diagnosed with Human Immunodeficiency Virus (HIV) or those who take immune-suppressing medications. The immune system can also work against itself in a condition referred to as autoimmune disease, which is discussed in the next section.

Many lifestyle factors that affect the immune system are within your control. Regular exercise, quality sleep, and certain foods can support and optimize immune defense. Chronic stress, lack of sleep, and malnutrition lower the body's ability to fight infection and disease. Alcohol, especially chronic alcohol abuse, can suppress the immune system. In addition, being either underweight or obese can lower the immune response in both children and adults.

AUTOIMMUNE DISEASE

Although the immune system works hard to protect the body from invaders, it can also work against you if it becomes overactive and begins attacking itself, creating chronic inflammation. This is what happens in autoimmune disease, which includes more than 80 chronic illnesses and affects more than 24 million Americans. Among the most well-known autoimmune diseases are type 1 diabetes, rheumatoid arthritis, multiple sclerosis, lupus, Sjögren syndrome, and Hashimoto's thyroiditis.

Nutrition plays an important role in autoimmune disease because certain foods can calm inflammation, reduce symptom flares, and help the body heal. Whole, minimally processed foods that are rich in antioxidants can be especially beneficial.

SUPPORTING THE IMMUNE SYSTEM THROUGH FOOD

Many macronutrients and micronutrients work together to support a strong immune system. The food you eat can absolutely make the difference. Vitamins A, C, D, and E as well as B vitamins, like folate and B_{12}, are critical parts of immune cells. Iron, selenium, and zinc each play unique roles in the immune system, too. Protein is an important foundation for enzymes and cells that are required to help the body fight infection and disease.

Whether a nutrient is needed for creating B cells (which mark invaders to create antibodies), T cells (which respond by recognizing and killing bacteria, viruses, and cancer cells), or the many enzymes that orchestrate this entire complex system, eating a variety of foods is important.

Certain foods have shown promise in creating a healthy immune response, whereas others can calm the chronic inflammation caused by autoimmune diseases. Studies have shown that some nutrients, namely vitamins, minerals, and antioxidants, including carotenoids and poly-phenols, can support immunity (Lange and Nakamura 2020). The nutrients that have also been shown to decrease inflammatory markers are found in many foods. For example, carrots, sweet potatoes, and tomatoes are high in carotenoids, and berries, cocoa, and beans are high in polyphenols. As an added bonus, many of these foods also contain fiber to help support a healthy gut microbiome.

What It All Means for Good Health

Now that you have a foundational understanding of the science behind the body's five major defense systems that Dr. Li establishes in *Eat to Beat Disease*, you can better understand the role food plays in optimizing how the body functions. You can also see the power that food has in fight-ing disease. Keeping the body in balance by providing the right types of nutrients is possible, and there's a lot of research to prove it. Next up is a discussion of exactly how to put it into practice in your life.

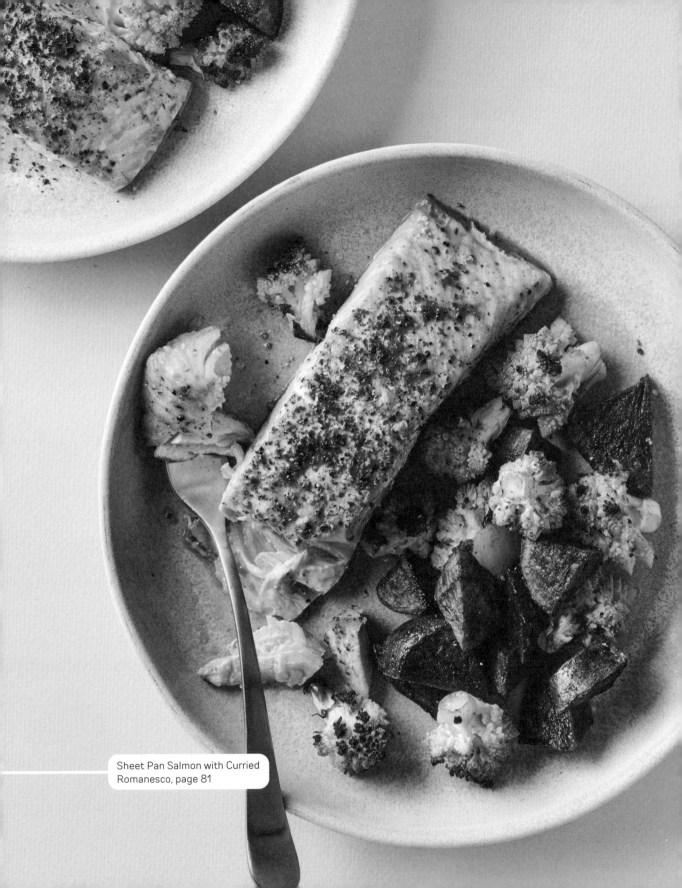

Sheet Pan Salmon with Curried
Romanesco, page 81

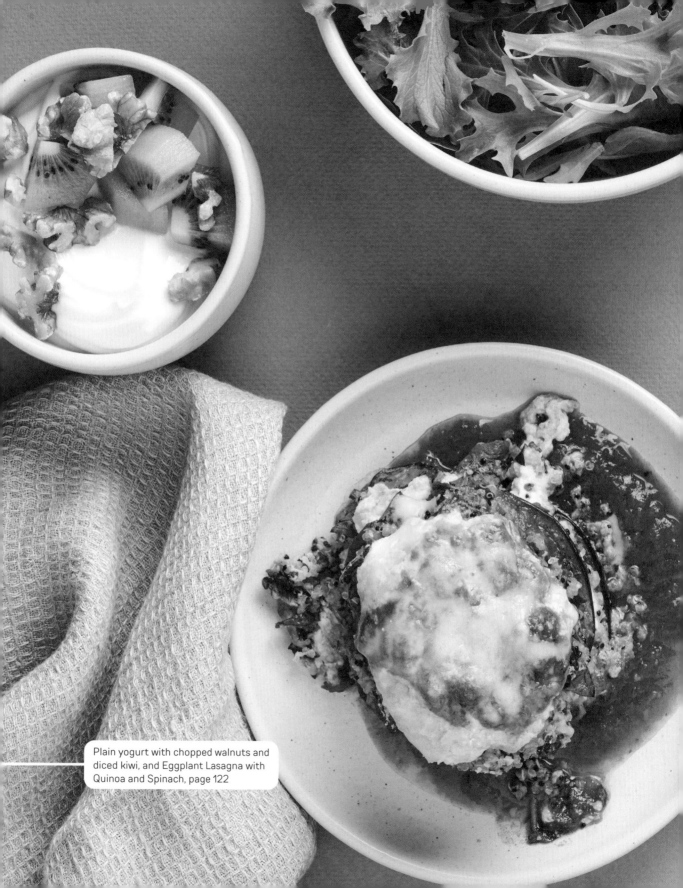

Plain yogurt with chopped walnuts and diced kiwi, and Eggplant Lasagna with Quinoa and Spinach, page 122

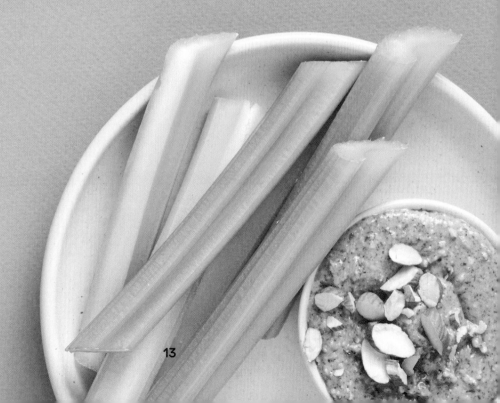

CHAPTER 2

How to Eat to Beat Disease and Stay Healthy

Now that you understand the five major defense systems and that certain foods can support their function, this chapter will provide the tools to make eating healthy a way of life. You'll get a comprehensive food list, specific strategies, and two full weeks of meal plans to provide structure and support.

Mindful Eating Every Day

Every time you eat, you make decisions that affect your health and can protect you from disease. Dr. Li developed a 5x5x5 plan, which is his easy way to get you to eat at least one food per day that supports each of the five defense systems. This plan is based on supporting the five defense systems by including at least five foods from the chart in meals and snacks, up to five times per day. It's about having a constant rotation of health-promoting foods you enjoy woven into your daily life.

You'll notice that most recipes have a wide variety of foods that support the five defense systems, so eating this way is a delicious and simple way to access many nutrients and health-boosting compounds. It is not meant to be prescriptive or restrictive but to open your horizons, showing you how many great-tasting options support your health goals.

As a registered dietitian, I want you to love food and have a good relationship with it. You can pick out the foods you enjoy and adjust recipes as appropriate for your dietary preferences and needs while using them and the structure provided here to create a long-term plan for you and your family.

SNACK SMART

The research on whether it's better to eat three square meals per day or smaller meals and more snacks is mixed (Hess, Jonnalagadda, and Slavin 2016). The best way to know what works for you is to listen to your personal hunger cues and assess your energy throughout the day. If you do choose to include a snack once or more per day, you have a lot of options to maximize health-promoting foods. There's no need to feel guilty about snacking; instead, use the snack suggestions in the meal plans in this chapter (page 30 and page 34) or the recipes in chapter 8 (page 137) to choose foods that have been shown to support the body's natural defense systems.

COOKING WITH PURPOSE

In the chapters that follow, you'll find 75 recipes, each of which contains at least two ingredients that have health-boosting and disease-fighting properties that fit into the *Eat to Beat Disease* concept. The recipes here do not include red meat (including pork, beef, etc.), because red meat doesn't often show up in the research or dietary patterns that appear to reduce the risk of chronic disease.

Use the food list to pick the foods you enjoy (no need to use them all), weaving them into meals that you already enjoy. You can pick the options that suit your tastes, are easy to find at your local markets, and fit within your budget.

Do No Harm

There are foods out there that do interfere with good health and are incompatible with a dietary pattern that's focused on preventing chronic disease. Regularly consuming foods like sugar-sweetened beverages, red meat (beef, lamb, pork), and processed meat (bacon, sausage, deli meat, hot dogs) has been shown consistently, across large studies, to be associated with increased risk of chronic diseases, including coronary heart disease, type 2 diabetes, some cancers, and stroke (Clark et al. 2019).

Saturated fat: Whether it's from high-fat dairy, meat, or even coconut oil, the current recommendations are to limit your intake of saturated fat to just 5% to 6% of your total calories. On a 2,000-calorie diet, that's about 13 grams per day. There are 4 grams in a teaspoon of butter or coconut oil.

Red and processed meat: Though the results of studies are mixed and the strength of the association between red and processed meat intake and increased risk of cancer, type 2 diabetes, and heart disease is still being assessed, it is clear that dietary patterns that include these foods regularly (i.e., the standard Western diet) do not protect against diseases as effectively as plant-based dietary patterns, such as vegetarian, vegan, and Mediterranean diets (Händel et al. 2019; Schwingshackl et al. 2016; Melina, Craig, and Levin 2016).

$\rightarrow$

Added sugar and artificial sweeteners: The guidelines on added sugar are clear—limit it to no more than 10% of your daily calories (200 calories or 12 teaspoons on a 2,000-calorie diet). According to the American Heart Association, Americans consume, on average, nearly 80 grams per day. An unprocessed, whole-food diet is naturally devoid of added sugars and sugar substitutes that are highly processed and do not contain beneficial fiber and antioxidants.

Excessive salt: An estimated 9 out of 10 Americans consume too much salt, and 70% of that comes directly from prepared, packaged, and restaurant foods. Eating too much salt is clearly linked in research to an increased risk of high blood pressure, which in turn can increase the risk of chronic diseases like heart attack, stroke, and heart failure. Reduce your salt intake to no more than 2,300 mg per day, and ideally no more than 1,500 mg per day, especially for adults with high blood pressure, which is easy to do if most of your foods are unprocessed.

Your Eat to Beat Disease Food List

This food list is organized alphabetically by food type. For each food, you can clearly see which defense systems it supports, so you can make the best choices for your individual goals and preferences.

INGREDIENT	ANGIOGENESIS	REGENERATION	MICROBIOME	DNA HEALTH	IMMUNE SYSTEM	ANGIOGENIC
FRUITS						
APPLE	•	•			•	Angiogenic and antiangiogenic
APRICOT	•		•	•	•	Antiangiogenic
AVOCADO			•			
BLACKBERRY	•	•		•	•	Antiangiogenic
BLUEBERRY	•	•	•	•	•	Antiangiogenic
CHERRY	•	•	•	•		Antiangiogenic
CRANBERRY	•	•	•		•	Antiangiogenic
GOJI BERRY		•			•	
GRAPE		•		•		
GRAPEFRUIT	•			•	•	Pink specifically is antiangiogenic because of the lycopene
GUAVA	•			•	•	Antiangiogenic
KIWI	•	•	•	•	•	Antiangiogenic
LEMON	•					Antiangiogenic
LYCHEE	•		•	•	•	Antiangiogenic
MANGO	•	•	•	•	•	Antiangiogenic
NECTARINE	•	•	•	•	•	Antiangiogenic
ORANGE				•	•	
PAPAYA				•		
PEACH	•	•	•	•	•	Antiangiogenic
PERSIMMON		•				
PLUM	•	•	•	•	•	Angiogenic and antiangiogenic
POMEGRANATE	•	•	•	•	•	Antiangiogenic

→

INGREDIENT	ANGIOGENESIS	REGENERATION	MICROBIOME	DNA HEALTH	IMMUNE SYSTEM	ANGIOGENIC
RAISIN	●	●			●	Angiogenic and antiangiogenic
RASPBERRY, RED AND BLACK	●	●			●	Antiangiogenic
STRAWBERRY	●	●		●	●	Antiangiogenic
WATERMELON	●			●		Antiangiogenic
VEGETABLES						
ARTICHOKE			●			
ARUGULA				●	●	
ASPARAGUS	●		●			Angiogenic
BEET			●			
BELGIAN ENDIVE	●	●			●	Angiogenic and antiangiogenic
BELL PEPPER					●	
BOK CHOY	●		●	●	●	Antiangiogenic
BROCCOLI	●		●	●	●	Antiangiogenic
BROCCOLI RABE	●			●	●	Antiangiogenic
BROCCOLI SPROUTS				●	●	
CABBAGE	●		●	●	●	Antiangiogenic
CARROT	●	●	●	●	●	Antiangiogenic
CAULIFLOWER	●		●	●	●	Antiangiogenic
CELERY	●	●				Antiangiogenic
CHILES	●	●	●		●	Antiangiogenic
COLLARD GREENS		●				
EGGPLANT	●	●	●	●	●	Antiangiogenic
ESCAROLE	●	●	●		●	Angiogenic and antiangiogenic
FIDDLEHEADS	●	●		●	●	Antiangiogenic

INGREDIENT	ANGIOGENESIS	REGENERATION	MICROBIOME	DNA HEALTH	IMMUNE SYSTEM	ANGIOGENIC
FRISÉE	●	●	●			Angiogenic
GREEN BEAN		●				
KALE	●		●	●	●	Antiangiogenic
LETTUCE, RED-LEAF	●	●				Angiogenic and antiangiogenic
MUSHROOM			●		●	
MUSTARD GREENS		●			●	
ONION	●	●			●	Antiangiogenic
PEAS			●			
POTATO, PURPLE		●				
RADICCHIO	●	●	●		●	Antiangiogenic
ROMANESCO				●	●	
RUTABAGA	●		●	●	●	Antiangiogenic
SPINACH					●	
SQUASH BLOSSOM	●	●		●	●	Antiangiogenic
SWEET POTATO					●	
SWISS CHARD		●			●	
TOMATO	●		●	●	●	Antiangiogenic
TRUFFLE		●		●	●	
TURNIP	●		●	●	●	Antiangiogenic
WATERCRESS		●			●	
HERBS & SPICES						
BASIL				●		
CINNAMON	●					Antiangiogenic
CUMIN	●				●	
GARLIC					●	
GINGER	●				●	Antiangiogenic
GINSENG	●	●			●	Angiogenic and antiangiogenic

→

INGREDIENT	ANGIOGENESIS	REGENERATION	MICROBIOME	DNA HEALTH	IMMUNE SYSTEM	ANGIOGENIC
LICORICE ROOT	•				•	Antiangiogenic
MARJORAM				•		
OREGANO	•	•				Antiangiogenic
PARSLEY	•					Antiangiogenic
PEPPERMINT	•	•		•	•	Angiogenic and antiangiogenic
ROSEMARY	•	•		•	•	Angiogenic and antiangiogenic
SAFFRON		•			•	
SAGE				•		
THYME		•		•		
TURMERIC	•	•		•	•	Antiangiogenic
WASABI		•				
NUTS & SEEDS						
ALMOND	•			•		Antiangiogenic
BRAZIL NUT				•		
CASHEW	•			•		Antiangiogenic
CHESTNUT				•	•	
CHIA SEED	•	•	•	•	•	Angiogenic and antiangiogenic
FLAXSEED	•	•	•	•	•	Angiogenic and antiangiogenic
HAZELNUT			•			
HEMPSEED			•			
MACADAMIA NUT	•			•		Antiangiogenic
PEANUT		•		•		
PECAN	•			•		Antiangiogenic
PINE NUT	•			•		Antiangiogenic
PISTACHIO	•	•		•		Antiangiogenic

INGREDIENT	ANGIOGENESIS	REGENERATION	MICROBIOME	DNA HEALTH	IMMUNE SYSTEM	ANGIOGENIC
PUMPKIN SEED	•	•	•	•	•	Angiogenic and antiangiogenic
SESAME SEED	•	•	•	•	•	Angiogenic and antiangiogenic
SOY NUT	•			•		Antiangiogenic
SUNFLOWER SEED	•	•	•	•		Angiogenic and antiangiogenic
WALNUT	•	•	•	•	•	Antiangiogenic
GRAINS & LEGUMES						
BARLEY	•	•			•	Angiogenic and antiangiogenic
BEANS (ALL KINDS: BLACK, NAVY, PINTO, KIDNEY, CHICKPEA, ETC.)	•		•			Antiangiogenic
BUCKWHEAT NOODLES	•				•	Antiangiogenic
EDAMAME	•		•	•		Antiangiogenic
LENTILS			•			
OATS			•		•	
QUINOA				•		
PUMPERNICKEL BREAD			•			
RICE, BROWN		•				
RYE			•			
TOFU	•			•		Antiangiogenic
WHOLE-WHEAT PASTA, FARRO, AND COUSCOUS		•	•			
FERMENTED FOODS						
CAPERS	•	•	•		•	Angiogenic and antiangiogenic
KIMCHI	•		•		•	Antiangiogenic
MISO			•	•		

→

INGREDIENT	ANGIOGENESIS	REGENERATION	MICROBIOME	DNA HEALTH	IMMUNE SYSTEM	ANGIOGENIC
SAUERKRAUT	•		•		•	Antiangiogenic
SOURDOUGH BREAD			•			
SOY SAUCE	•		•	•		Antiangiogenic
TEMPEH	•		•	•		Antiangiogenic
YOGURT			•			
CHEESE						
CAMEMBERT	•		•			Antiangiogenic
EDAM	•		•			Antiangiogenic
EMMENTHAL/SWISS CHEESE	•		•			Antiangiogenic
GOUDA	•		•			Antiangiogenic
JARLSBERG	•		•			Antiangiogenic
MUENSTER	•		•			Antiangiogenic
PARMIGIANO-REGGIANO	•		•			Antiangiogenic
STILTON	•		•			Antiangiogenic
SEAFOOD						
ANCHOVY	•	•		•		Antiangiogenic
ARCTIC CHAR	•	•		•		Antiangiogenic
BLACK BASS	•	•		•		Antiangiogenic
BLUEFISH	•	•		•		Antiangiogenic
BOTTARGA	•	•		•		Antiangiogenic
CAVIAR (STURGEON) AND FISH ROE (SALMON)	•	•		•		Antiangiogenic
CLAMS, COCKLES AND MANILA	•	•		•	•	Antiangiogenic
HAKE	•	•		•		Antiangiogenic
HALIBUT	•	•		•		Antiangiogenic
LOBSTER, SPINY	•	•		•		Antiangiogenic
MACKEREL	•	•		•		Antiangiogenic
MULLET, GRAY AND RED	•	•		•		Antiangiogenic

INGREDIENT	ANGIOGENESIS	REGENERATION	MICROBIOME	DNA HEALTH	IMMUNE SYSTEM	ANGIOGENIC
OYSTER, EASTERN AND PACIFIC	●	●		●	●	Antiangiogenic
POMPANO	●	●		●		Antiangiogenic
RAINBOW TROUT	●	●		●		Antiangiogenic
REDFISH	●	●		●		Antiangiogenic
SALMON	●	●		●		Antiangiogenic
SARDINE	●	●		●		Antiangiogenic
SEA BREAM	●	●		●		Antiangiogenic
SQUID INK	●	●		●		Antiangiogenic
TUNA, BIGEYE, BLUEFIN, YELLOWTAIL	●	●		●		Antiangiogenic
MEAT						
CHICKEN (DARK MEAT)	●					Antiangiogenic
PANTRY ITEMS						
CHOCOLATE, DARK (COCOA AND CACAO)		●	●		●	
OLIVE OIL, EXTRA-VIRGIN	●	●	●		●	Antiangiogenic
TAHINI				●		
BEVERAGES						
BEER	●	●	●			Antiangiogenic
COFFEE	●	●	●	●	●	Antiangiogenic
CONCORD GRAPE JUICE		●	●	●	●	
CRANBERRY JUICE			●		●	
ORANGE JUICE				●	●	
POMEGRANATE JUICE			●			
RED WINE	●	●	●	●	●	Antiangiogenic
SOY MILK	●			●		Antiangiogenic
TEA (BLACK, GREEN, CHAMOMILE)	●	●	●	●	●	Antiangiogenic
WHITE WINE	●	●	●	●		Antiangiogenic

Drink to Your Health!

Beverages, some alcoholic and some not, have been linked in studies to a variety of health-promoting benefits, including antiangiogenic effects, a healthy microbiome, and even stem cell regeneration and DNA protection. These drinks have unique antioxidants that contribute to their protective benefits. Though water should be your main beverage every day for hydration, including low to moderate amounts of red wine and beer, if you consume alcohol, as well as coffee, tea, and some juices can benefit your health goals.

RED WINE

There is a large volume of human research showing red wine's benefits, including reduced cardiovascular risk, a healthy gut microbiome, and even a reduced risk of colorectal cancer. Keep in mind that many studies finding health benefits are based on small amounts of red wine, some as little as about half a glass per day. As intake increases, the health benefits disappear and are replaced with poorer outcomes and a higher risk of many diseases.

BEER

Beer is not only antiangiogenic and stem cell boosting but also contains unique antioxidants and even some vitamins and minerals. Like wine, it's a fermented product, which could be the reason behind its positive health outcomes when consumed at low levels. Studies have shown its potential for reducing the risk of some cancers and lowering the risk of cardiac disease (De Gaetano et al. 2016). With all alcohol, studies show that moderate amounts that follow national guidelines may be beneficial; a serving of beer is 12 ounces. As in the case of wine, as intake increases, so do the negative health outcomes.

BLACK, GREEN, AND CHAMOMILE TEA

Packed full of bioactive compounds (including the potent epigallocatechin-3-gallate [EGCG] in green tea), tea has been found to have antiangiogenic, stem cell–boosting, microbiome-supporting, and even DNA-protecting effects (Mitra and Khandelwal 2017). Studies show that green, black, and herbal teas, including chamomile, may be beneficial in helping reduce the risk of diabetes and heart disease and even potentially reducing cancer risk by boosting a powerful antioxidant enzyme that supports detoxification, called glutathione-S-transferase (GSTP1) (Altay et al. 2017). Tea is also hydrating, comforting, and even stress relieving, so include it daily as one of your staple beverages, aside from plain water.

COFFEE

There is good evidence that coffee has many health benefits and can support the body's defenses, especially counteracting telomere shortening and protecting DNA (Fang, Chen, and Yang 2007). The potent antioxidants in coffee beans, chlorogenic and caffeic acids, have the ability to turn on RARB2, a tumor-suppressing gene. These antioxidants exhibit anti-inflammatory effects and have been tied to blood sugar regulation, reduction of cardiovascular disease risk, weight control, and even some anticancer benefits (Tajik et al. 2017). Large, human studies have shown that drinking both caffeinated and decaffeinated coffee is associated with reduced mortality in men and women, including reduced risk of death from digestive-related diseases (Gunter et al. 2017).

Think beyond Food to Really Beat Disease

All the kale or blueberries in the world can't help you optimize your health if you're not taking a holistic approach and supporting your body in many different ways. Here are some other ways to boost your body's natural ability to ward off disease:

Exercise

Being physically active is well known for its cardiovascular, blood sugar–regulating, and anticancer benefits, but it also affects the body's defense systems. Angiogenesis occurs when exercise places stress on your bones; this is the reason that exercise helps make bones stronger. There is also a direct connection between moderate exercise and a well-functioning immune system. Studies have even shown that exercise, especially resistance training, can help protect DNA by improving the activity of the telomerase enzyme.

Current guidelines tell us that getting at least 150 to 300 minutes per week of moderate-intensity activity like brisk walking or 75 to 150 minutes of vigorous-intensity aerobic activity like running (or a combination of both) and two or more days per week of resistance training that works all the major muscle groups can help optimize health and avoid chronic disease (Fiorenza et al. 2020; Hooshmand-Moghadam et al. 2020).

Sleep

Getting enough undisturbed sleep is actually linked to a longer life expectancy, with the best outcomes in studies for those who sleep 7 to 8½ hours per night. There is a direct link between getting enough sleep and the immune system functioning properly. Research shows that those who get less than 6 hours of sleep per night are more vulnerable to viral infections and even respond less well to vaccinations designed to launch immune responses against certain diseases, including influenza. Sleep may even play a role in a healthy microbiome; better sleep could equal a more diverse array of bacteria in the gut (Smith et al. 2019).

Stress Management

Chronic stress can damage the body and hurt your health. In a study of long-term caregivers, those who had better resilience to the stress of taking care of others actually had less shortening of their telomeres than those with more stress (Mason et al. 2019). Stress can decrease the functioning of the immune system over time; chronic stress causes elevated hormone levels (cortisol), which can depress immunity. There's even evidence that stress can increase inflammation in the gut, harming your microbiome (Peirce and Alviña 2019).

The links between foods that support the body's defense systems and lifestyle factors like exercise, sleep, and stress cannot be ignored. Be sure to take a holistic approach to your health when you think about beating disease long term.

Getting Started with a Meal Plan

These two meal plans are each one week long, and each includes a shopping list for the week's recipes. The meal plans are put together as a guide that will show you how you can easily incorporate foods that support the five major defense systems on a day-to-day basis. A variety of breakfast, snack, lunch, and dinner recipes from the book are included, as well as some raw foods, eaten on their own, so you can get the full coverage of health benefits every day.

Some ingredients and recipes are reused to reduce both your prep time and potential food waste. You may see a breakfast recipe show up as a snack the following day or later that week or leftovers from a dinner entrée used as a lunch the next day. This is an example of how you can plan out your weeks to maximize your intake of a variety of healthy food but minimize the time you spend in the kitchen doing food prep. Feel free to swap in recipes that you prefer or adjust the plan for your dietary needs or allergies. You can easily make each plan simpler or more complex based on your unique lifestyle.

SHOPPING LIST FOR WEEK 1

CANNED ITEMS

→ Beans, white
  (1 [15-ounce] can)

→ Chickpeas
  (1 [15-ounce] can)

→ Coconut milk, light
  (1 [13½-ounce] can)

→ Stock, vegetable
  (1 [32-ounce]
  container)

DRIED HERBS & SPICES

→ Chili powder

→ Coriander, ground

→ Cumin, ground

→ Curry powder

→ Oregano

→ Peppercorns, black

→ Red pepper flakes

→ Rosemary

→ Salt

→ Turmeric

PANTRY

→ Almond butter

→ Almonds, roasted
  unsalted or raw

→ Baking powder

→ Baking soda

→ Bread, sourdough
  (or if homemade,
  include ingredients
  on page 140)

→ Cacao or
  cocoa powder,
  unsweetened

→ Coffee

→ Flour, all-purpose

- → Hempseed
- → Honey
- → Lentils, dried, red
- → Maple syrup
- → Miso
- → Mustard, Dijon
- → Oats, rolled (make sure to check for gluten-free if you have a wheat allergy)
- → Oil, olive
- → Oil, olive, extra-virgin
- → Oil, vegetable
- → Quinoa
- → Rice, brown
- → Sourdough starter (or if homemade, include ingredients on page 138)
- → Soy sauce, low-sodium
- → Sugar
- → Tahini
- → Vanilla extract, pure
- → Vinegar, apple cider
- → Vinegar, red wine

PRODUCE

- → Avocados (2)
- → Bananas (2 medium)
- → Basil (1 bunch)
- → Bell peppers (2 medium)
- → Blueberries, fresh or frozen (1 pint or 1 [10-ounce] bag)
- → Bok choy, baby (2 pounds)
- → Broccoli (1 small head)
- → Brussels sprouts (1 pound)
- → Carrots (3 large)
- → Cauliflower (1 medium head, 2 small heads)
- → Celery (1 bunch)
- → Cilantro (2 bunches)
- → Cucumbers (2)
- → Dill (1 bunch)
- → Garlic (2 heads)
- → Ginger (1)
- → Jalapeños (3)
- → Lemon (1)
- → Lettuce, red-leaf (1 head)
- → Limes (3)
- → Mint (1 bunch)
- → Mushrooms (1 pound)
- → Peaches (2)
- → Potatoes, purple (1½ pounds)
- → Onion, red (1 small)
- → Onions, yellow (1 large, 2 small)
- → Oranges (3 large)
- → Raspberries, fresh or frozen, red or black (1 pint or 1 [10-ounce] bag)
- → Romanesco (1 head)
- → Spinach (1 bunch)
- → Tomatoes, cherry (1 pint)
- → Turmeric root (1)
- → Watercress (1 [5-ounce] bag)

PROTEIN

- → Chicken, thighs, bone-in, skin-on (8 small)
- → Eggs (½ dozen)
- → Hummus (1 [8-ounce] container)
- → Salmon, skin-on (4 [4-ounce] fillets)
- → Trout (4 [4-ounce] fillets)

DAIRY & DAIRY ALTERNATIVES

- → Soy milk, unsweetened (½ gallon)
- → Yogurt, Greek, plain (32 ounces)

Meal Plan Week 1

MEAL	MON	TUES	WEDS
BREAKFAST	Mocha Smoothie with Almond Butter (page 38)	Sourdough Avocado Toast with Hempseed (page 44)	Peaches and Cream Oatmeal (page 42)
LUNCH	Creamy Mushroom Soup (page 63) with sourdough bread (see page 140)	Tomato-Basil White Bean and Quinoa Salad (page 57)	Leftover Garlic Chickpea Bowls with Miso-Tahini Dressing topped with leftover salmon
SNACK	An orange and a handful of almonds	Leftover Mocha Smoothie with Almond Butter	Celery with almond butter
DINNER	Garlic Chickpea Bowls with Miso-Tahini Dressing (page 124)	Sheet Pan Salmon with Curried Romanesco (page 81) with Simple Greens with Apple Cider Vinegar Dressing (page 56)	Leftover Creamy Mushroom Soup with sourdough bread (see page 140) and leftover Simple Greens with Apple Cider Vinegar Dressing

THURS	FRI	SAT	SUN
Berry Yogurt Parfait with Almonds (page 41)	Leftover Sourdough Avocado Toast with Hempseed	Fluffy Sourdough Pancakes (page 45)	Savory Vegetable Breakfast Skillet (page 46)
Leftover Tomato-Basil White Bean and Quinoa Salad	Leftover Sheet Pan Citrus Chicken with Brussels Sprouts	Leftover Red Lentil Curry with Cauliflower	Leftover Trout with Yogurt-Dill Sauce with a side of leftover Garlic Bok Choy
Broccoli and cauliflower florets with hummus	Leftover Berry Yogurt Parfait with Almonds	Cucumber slices with hummus	Carrot with almond butter
Sheet Pan Citrus Chicken with Brussels Sprouts (page 104)	Red Lentil Curry with Cauliflower (page 132)	Trout with Yogurt-Dill Sauce (page 79) with a side of Garlic Bok Choy (page 113)	Leftover Sheet Pan Citrus Chicken with Brussels Sprouts

SHOPPING LIST FOR WEEK 2

CANNED ITEMS

→ Artichoke hearts
(1 [15-ounce] can)

→ Beans, pinto
(1 [15-ounce] can)

→ Beans, white
(4 [15½-ounce] cans)

→ Coconut milk, light
(1 [13½-ounce] can)

→ Marinara sauce
(1 [26-ounce] jar)

→ Olives, Kalamata
(1 [8-ounce] jar)

→ Salmon
(2 [5-ounce] cans)

→ Stock, vegetable
(2 [32-ounce]
containers)

DRIED HERBS & SPICES

→ Basil

→ Chili powder

→ Cinnamon, ground

→ Cumin, ground

→ Curry powder

→ Dill

→ Ginger, ground

→ Oregano

→ Parsley

→ Peppercorns, black

→ Rosemary

→ Salt

→ Salt, sea

→ Turmeric

PANTRY

→ Almond butter

→ Baking powder

→ Baking soda

→ Bread crumbs,
panko, whole-wheat

→ Bread, sourdough
(or if homemade,
include ingredients
on page 140)

→ Cashews, whole,
roasted unsalted

→ Chia seeds

→ Flaxseed, ground

→ Flour, all-purpose

→ Hazelnuts

→ Honey

→ Maple syrup

→ Mustard, Dijon

→ Oats, rolled

→ Oil, olive,
extra-virgin

→ Oil, vegetable

→ Penne, whole-wheat
or bean (12 ounces)

→ Pine nuts

→ Quinoa

→ Rice, brown

→ Sourdough starter
(or if homemade,

include ingredients
on page 138)

→ Sugar

→ Tahini

→ Tea, green

→ Vanilla extract, pure

→ Vinegar, apple cider

→ Vinegar, white wine

→ Walnuts,
whole, roasted
unsalted or raw

→ Wine, white

PRODUCE

→ Asparagus
(1 pound)

→ Banana (1 medium)

→ Basil (1 bunch)

→ Bell peppers (7)

→ Blueberries, fresh
or frozen (1 pint or
1 [10-ounce] bag)

→ Carrots (4)

→ Cauliflower
(1 small head)

→ Celery (1 bunch)

→ Chives (1 bunch)

→ Cucumber (1)

→ Dill (1 bunch)

→ Eggplants
(2 medium)

→ Garlic (2 heads)

→ Ginger (1)

→ Jalapeño (1)

→ Kale (2 bunches)

→ Kiwis (2)

→ Lemons (3)

→ Lettuce, red-leaf
(2 heads)

→ Mangos (2 large
or 1 bag)

→ Mushrooms
(24, plus
1 [8-ounce] package)

→ Onions, yellow (4)

→ Parsley (1 bunch)

→ Raspberries, red
or black, fresh or
frozen (1 pint or
1 [10-ounce] bag)

→ Scallions (1 bunch)

→ Spinach (1 bunch)

→ Spinach, baby
(1 [5-ounce] bag)

→ Thyme (1 bunch)

→ Tomato (1)

→ Zucchini (1)

PROTEIN

→ Chicken, thighs,
boneless, skinless
(1½ pounds)

→ Eggs (½ dozen)

→ Hummus
(1 [8-ounce]
container)

→ Salmon (1 pound)

→ Tofu, firm
(1 [12-ounce]
package)

→ Tofu, extra-firm
silken (1 [12-ounce]
package)

DAIRY (DAIRY ALTERNATIVES ARE FINE FOR ALL)

→ Cheese, Gouda
(6 ounces)

→ Cheese, mozzarella
(1 [8-ounce] ball)

→ Cheese,
Parmigiano-
Reggiano
(6 ounces)

→ Cheese, ricotta
(1 [8-ounce]
container)

→ Soy milk,
unsweetened
(½ gallon)

→ Yogurt, Greek,
plain (1 [5-ounce]
container)

→ Yogurt, plain
(12 ounces)

Meal Plan Week 2

MEAL	MON	TUES	WEDS
BREAKFAST	Raspberry, Ginger, and Hazelnut Chia Pudding (page 152)	High-Protein Green Tea Smoothie (page 39)	Cinnamon-Walnut Oat Bake (page 43)
LUNCH	Savory Vegetarian Navy Bean Soup (page 53) with Kale Caesar with Parmigiano-Reggiano and Homemade Croutons (page 60)	Leftover Savory Vegetarian Navy Bean Soup with Simple Greens with Apple Cider Vinegar Dressing (page 56)	Leftover Eggplant Lasagna with Quinoa and Spinach
SNACK	Carrot sticks with hummus	Leftover Raspberry, Ginger, and Hazelnut Chia Pudding	Leftover High-Protein Green Tea Smoothie
DINNER	Lemon-Thyme Salmon Meatballs (page 74) over rice with Savory Roasted Cauliflower (page 114)	Eggplant Lasagna with Quinoa and Spinach (page 122) with leftover Kale Caesar with Parmigiano-Reggiano and Homemade Croutons	Leftover Lemon-Thyme Salmon Meatballs over rice with leftover Savory Roasted Cauliflower

THURS	FRI	SAT	SUN
Plain yogurt with chopped walnuts and diced kiwi	Leftover Cinnamon-Walnut Oat Bake	Mushroom and Tofu Scramble (page 47)	Fluffy Sourdough Pancakes (page 45) with berries
Herb-Stuffed Mushrooms (page 116) with leftover Simple Greens with Apple Cider Vinegar Dressing	Leftover Chicken in Mango-Cashew Curry over rice	Leftover Penne with Pesto and Antipasti	5-Minute Salmon Salad (page 65)
Leftover Cinnamon-Walnut Oat Bake	Leftover Herb-Stuffed Mushrooms	Plain yogurt with chopped walnuts and diced kiwi	Celery with almond butter
Chicken in Mango-Cashew Curry (page 96) over rice with a green garden salad	Penne with Pesto and Antipasti (page 134) with a green garden salad	Leftover Chicken in Mango-Cashew Curry with Citrus-Herb Asparagus (page 115)	Vegetarian Stuffed Bell Peppers (page 120)

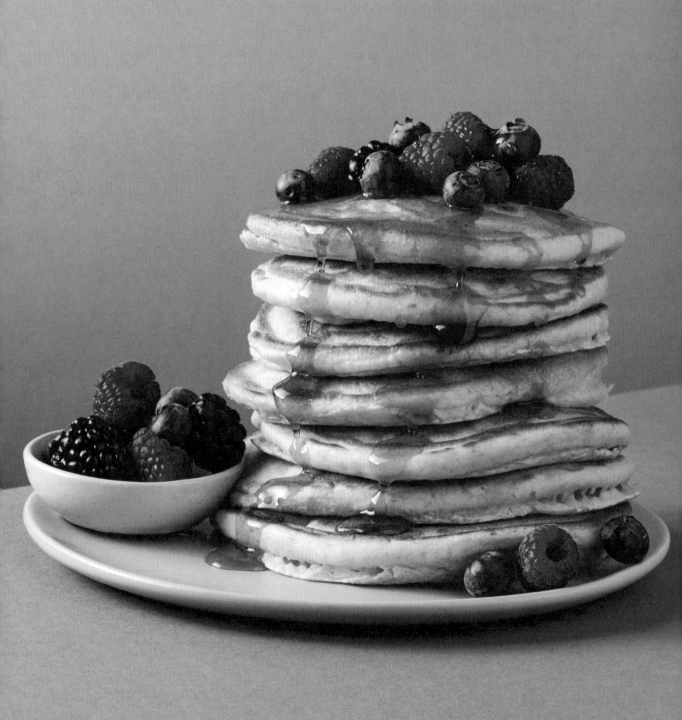

CHAPTER 3

Breakfast

The first meal of the day is the perfect opportunity to fuel up with health-promoting foods that support all five defense systems. Breakfast should be an easy, delicious meal that you look forward to. Whether you enjoy a sweet or savory start to your day, there are options here for you, and all of these recipes are simple and plant based. Whip up a smoothie, grab an energy ball or parfait on the go, or take your time with some pancakes or a savory breakfast skillet.

Mocha Smoothie with Almond Butter

Dairy-Free, Gluten-Free,
Vegan

SERVES 2

PREP TIME: 5 MINUTES

Enjoy your coffee in a new way, blended in a delicious smoothie without any added sugar whatsoever. This morning beverage is perfectly balanced with protein and healthy fat from the almond butter and plenty of antioxidant-rich compounds that support all five defense systems.

1 cup brewed coffee, chilled in the refrigerator

1 frozen medium banana, peeled

1 cup unsweetened soy milk

1 cup ice

½ tablespoon unsweetened cacao powder or unsweetened cocoa powder

1 tablespoon almond butter

1 teaspoon vanilla extract

Bioactive ingredients: coffee, soy milk, cacao, almond butter

In a blender, combine the coffee, banana, soy milk, ice, cacao powder, almond butter, and vanilla. Blend for 30 to 60 seconds, or until smooth. Store in the refrigerator for up to 48 hours, then add 2 or 3 new ice cubes, blend again, and enjoy when you're ready.

Per Serving: Calories: 147; Total fat: 6g; Saturated fat: 1g; Protein: 5g; Total carbohydrates: 20g; Fiber: 3g; Sugar: 11g; Cholesterol: 0g

→ **VARIATION:** If you like your smoothies sweeter, adjust the amount of banana to suit your preference. You can also add more cacao or cocoa, if desired, for added antioxidants and chocolate flavor. You can use other types of nondairy milk, but you will lose some of the health benefits of the soy milk.

High-Protein Green Tea Smoothie

Gluten-Free, Nut-Free,
Soy-Free, Vegetarian

SERVES 2

PREP TIME: 10 MINUTES

This beautiful purple smoothie combines high-fiber, filling ingredients as well as yogurt and chia seeds for protein. Using green tea as the base for your smoothie adds unique health benefits, a vibrant flavor, and lots of antioxidants. If you don't drink caffeine, consider a decaffeinated green tea instead.

1 green tea bag

1½ cups boiling water

1 frozen medium banana, peeled

½ cup frozen blueberries

½ cup baby spinach

3 ounces nonfat plain yogurt or soy yogurt

1 tablespoon ground flaxseed

1 teaspoon chia seeds

1 cup ice cubes, divided

Bioactive ingredients: green tea, blueberry, spinach, yogurt, flaxseed, chia seed

1. Put the green tea bag in a large, heatproof measuring cup.

2. Add the water. Steep for 1 to 2 minutes, or until the tea reaches your desired strength.

3. While the tea steeps, put the banana, blueberries, spinach, yogurt, flaxseed, and chia seeds in a blender.

4. Drop ½ cup of ice cubes into the tea to cool it partially. Pour into the blender, and add the remaining ½ cup of ice cubes. Blend for about 1 minute, or until smooth.

Per Serving: Calories: 125; Total fat: 4g; Saturated fat: 1g; Protein: 3g; Total carbohydrates: 22g; Fiber: 4g; Sugar: 13g; Cholesterol: 6g

→ **VARIATION:** Increase the chia seeds to 2 teaspoons and/or the flaxseed to 2 tablespoons to double your fiber intake. Make sure to grind your flaxseed, because that's the way the body is best able to absorb its benefits.

Apricot Energy Balls

Dairy-Free, Gluten-Free,
Soy-Free, Vegetarian

SERVES 12 (24 BALLS)

PREP TIME: 10 MINUTES, PLUS 1 HOUR TO SET

Having a quick, easy breakfast or snack on hand makes eating healthy easier. These no-bake energy balls are packed with fiber, vitamins, minerals, and antioxidants to support the immune system and gut microbiome. They are perfect for busy mornings and are balanced with dried fruit, nuts, and rich tahini.

1½ cups dried apricots

1 cup unsalted cashews

¾ cup rolled oats

½ cup finely shredded, unsweetened coconut

5 tablespoons tahini

2 tablespoons honey

¾ teaspoon grated fresh ginger

⅛ teaspoon salt

Bioactive ingredients: apricot, cashew, oats, tahini, ginger

1. Put the apricots, cashews, oats, and coconut in a food processor. Pulse about 20 times, or until the nuts and apricots are finely chopped and crumbly.

2. Add the tahini, honey, ginger, and salt. Process on high speed for 1 minute, or until the mixture sticks together and starts to form a ball.

3. Using your clean hands, shape 1 tablespoon of the dough into a bite-size ball. Repeat until all of the dough has been used.

4. Place the balls in a storage container, cover, and refrigerate for about 1 hour, or until the balls have set. Store in the refrigerator for up to 5 days or in the freezer for up to 2 months.

Per Serving: Calories: 195; Total fat: 10g; Saturated fat: 3g; Protein: 5g; Total carbohydrates: 24g; Fiber: 3g; Sugar: 12g; Cholesterol: 0g

→ **VARIATION:** You can swap out the dried apricots for the same portion of unsweetened dried cherries or blueberries. If your cashews are salted, eliminate the ⅛ teaspoon salt. Make this recipe vegan by using maple syrup or agave instead of honey.

Berry Yogurt Parfait with Almonds

Gluten-Free, Soy-Free, Vegetarian

SERVES 2

PREP TIME: 5 MINUTES

Fitting in a healthy breakfast on the go is a breeze when you plan ahead. Consider making these parfaits ahead of time in Mason jars with lids so you can grab one for breakfast or a snack as you leave the house in the morning.

2 cups nonfat plain Greek yogurt or soy yogurt

½ cup fresh or frozen red or black raspberries

½ cup fresh or frozen blueberries

½ cup raw or roasted unsalted sliced almonds

2 teaspoons maple syrup

Bioactive ingredients: yogurt, red or black raspberry, blueberry, almond

1. Layer the yogurt, raspberries, blueberries, and almonds into 2 bowls, glasses, or jars.
2. Drizzle the maple syrup on top.

Per Serving: Calories: 353; Total fat: 15g; Saturated fat: 2g; Protein: 31g; Total carbohydrates: 28g; Fiber: 7g; Sugar: 18g; Cholesterol: 11g

→ **VARIATION:** Swap out the almonds for other nuts, such as chopped walnuts, cashews, hazelnuts, or pecans. Or add in some chia, hempseed, or ground flaxseed for added health benefits. Other berries can be added or swapped in as well; consider strawberries, goji berries, blackberries, or even pomegranate arils.

Peaches and Cream Oatmeal

Dairy-Free, Gluten-Free, Nut-Free, Vegan	**SERVES 2** PREP TIME: 5 MINUTES / COOK TIME: 10 MINUTES

A bowl of hot oats will start your day off right with a health-supporting combination of ingredients. Packed with fiber as well as flavor, this comforting meal can be enjoyed year-round by substituting frozen or canned peaches (in their own juice or no sugar added) for the fresh peaches.

2 cups unsweetened soy milk

1 cup rolled oats

½ peeled frozen medium banana

1 cup chopped peeled fresh peaches

Bioactive ingredients: soy milk, oats, peach

1. In a medium saucepan, combine the milk and oats. Bring to a boil over medium-high heat.

2. Add the banana.

3. Reduce the heat to low. Simmer for 3 to 5 minutes, or until the oats have thickened and the banana is soft.

4. Using a potato masher or a fork, mix the banana into the oats until fully incorporated.

5. Add the peaches, then stir to combine. Remove from the heat. Serve hot.

Per Serving: Calories: 342; Total fat: 6g; Saturated fat: 1g; Protein: 16g; Total carbohydrates: 59g; Fiber: 8g; Sugar: 16g; Cholesterol: 0g

→ **VARIATION:** Add chopped walnuts, flaxseed, or both for a boost to all five defense systems plus anti-inflammatory omega-3 essential fatty acids and more protein. For added sweetness, use a whole banana instead of half.

Cinnamon-Walnut Oat Bake

Dairy-Free, Gluten-Free,
Vegetarian

SERVES 9

PREP TIME: 10 MINUTES / COOK TIME: 30 MINUTES,
PLUS 30 MINUTES TO COOL

You don't need a stovetop to make a delicious oatmeal breakfast. Pop this one in the oven while getting ready in the morning for a hands-off breakfast option. Comforting flavors like cinnamon, vanilla, and maple syrup brighten the oats, while walnuts add health benefits and a crunchy texture.

1 teaspoon extra-virgin olive oil

1 egg

1⅓ cups unsweetened soy milk

¼ cup maple syrup

1 teaspoon pure vanilla extract

½ teaspoon ground cinnamon

¼ teaspoon sea salt

3 cups rolled oats

1 cup walnuts

Bioactive ingredients: soy milk, cinnamon, oats, walnut

1. Preheat the oven to 375°F. Brush an 8-by-8-inch square glass baking dish with the oil.

2. In a large mixing bowl, beat the egg.

3. Add the soy milk, maple syrup, vanilla, cinnamon, and salt. Using a wooden spoon, mix together.

4. Stir in the oats, then fold in the walnuts until they are evenly distributed throughout the batter.

5. Spread the batter in the prepared baking dish.

6. Transfer the baking dish to the oven, and bake for 30 to 40 minutes, or until the top is a light toasty brown. Remove from the oven. Let cool for about 30 minutes before slicing and serving. Store leftovers, covered, in the refrigerator for up to 5 days.

Per Serving: Calories: 292; Total fat: 13g; Saturated fat: 2g; Protein: 10g; Total carbohydrates: 36g; Fiber: 5g; Sugar: 7g; Cholesterol: 18g

Sourdough Avocado Toast with Hempseed

Dairy-Free, Nut-Free, Soy-Free, Vegan	**SERVES 2** PREP TIME: 5 MINUTES / COOK TIME: 3 MINUTES

Avocado toast is packed full of fiber and healthy fat from everyone's favorite savory fruit. You can boost the health benefits even more by pairing it with gut-supporting homemade (page 140) or store-bought sourdough bread and topping it with hempseed for both protein and anti-inflammatory omega-3 fatty acids.

2 large sourdough bread slices

1 medium ripe avocado

¼ teaspoon salt

2 teaspoons freshly squeezed lemon juice

1 tablespoon hempseed

½ cup watercress

Bioactive ingredients: sourdough bread, avocado, lemon, hempseed

1. Toast the bread in the toaster for 2 to 3 minutes. Transfer to a plate.

2. While the bread is toasting, cut the avocado in half, and remove the pit. Using a spoon, scoop the flesh out into a small mixing bowl.

3. Add the salt and lemon juice. Using a fork, mash together until well combined.

4. Spread the avocado mixture evenly onto each slice of toast.

5. Sprinkle with the hempseed, and top with the watercress.

Per Serving: Calories: 373; Total fat: 17g; Saturated fat: 3g; Protein: 11g; Total carbohydrates: 49g; Fiber: 10g; Sugar: 6g; Cholesterol: 0g

→ **VARIATION:** If you don't have hempseed, any other type of small nut or seed can be substituted in the same amount. Consider chia, pine nuts, chopped pumpkin seeds, or sesame seeds for different flavors and health benefits. You could replace the watercress with the same amount of arugula or chopped spinach if desired.

Fluffy Sourdough Pancakes

Dairy-Free, Nut-Free, Vegetarian

SERVES 4 (12 MEDIUM PANCAKES)

PREP TIME: 10 MINUTES / COOK TIME: 10 MINUTES

Pancakes get a microbiome-benefiting boost when they're made with sourdough starter. Plus, they'll have a slightly tangy flavor that adds more complexity to your typical breakfast. Serve these pancakes with fresh or cooked berries or no-sugar-added jam instead of traditional maple syrup for even more disease-fighting benefits.

1¾ cups all-purpose flour

2 tablespoons sugar

2 teaspoons baking powder

1 teaspoon baking soda

½ teaspoon salt

1½ cups unsweetened soy milk

1 egg

2 tablespoons vegetable oil, plus more for greasing

½ teaspoon pure vanilla extract

1 cup Sourdough Starter (page 138)

Bioactive ingredients: soy milk, sourdough

1. In a large bowl, combine the flour, sugar, baking powder, baking soda, and salt.

2. In a small mixing bowl, whisk together the soy milk, egg, oil, and vanilla.

3. Add the sourdough starter to the small bowl, and stir using a wooden spoon until well combined.

4. Pour the wet mixture into the dry mixture, and stir well.

5. Preheat a pancake griddle or a large skillet, then grease lightly with oil.

6. In ¼-cup portions, pour the batter onto the hot griddle. Cook for 2 to 3 minutes, or until the pancakes are bubbling thoroughly on the top.

7. Flip the pancakes, and cook for 1 to 2 minutes, or until they have risen. Remove from the heat. Serve hot.

Per Serving: Calories: 460; Total fat: 11g; Saturated fat: 2g; Protein: 14g; Total carbohydrates: 78g; Fiber: 4g; Sugar: 10g; Cholesterol: 41g

Savory Vegetable Breakfast Skillet

Dairy-Free, Gluten-Free,
Nut-Free, Soy-Free, Vegan

SERVES 2–4

PREP TIME: 30 MINUTES, PLUS 20 MINUTES
TO SOAK / COOK TIME: 25 MINUTES

This skillet is the ultimate way to increase the number of disease-fighting vegetables in your breakfast. This recipe is designed to be egg-free, with seasoned cauliflower serving as the base. The great news is that, like most recipes in this book, it's versatile, so if you'd like to add eggs, feel free.

2 tablespoons extra-virgin olive oil

8 ounces purple potatoes, chopped and soaked in water for 20 minutes, then drained and patted dry (about 3 to 4 potatoes)

1 small yellow onion, chopped

2 medium bell peppers, seeded and chopped

1 medium head cauliflower, cut into bite-size florets

3 garlic cloves, minced

½ teaspoon salt

½ teaspoon freshly ground black pepper

1 teaspoon turmeric

Bioactive ingredients: purple potato, onion, bell pepper, cauliflower, garlic, turmeric

1. In a medium skillet, heat the oil over medium-high heat.

2. Add the potatoes, and sauté, stirring occasionally, for 10 minutes, or until beginning to soften. Add water, 1 tablespoon at a time, if needed to prevent sticking.

3. Add the onion, peppers, and cauliflower. Cook for 7 to 9 minutes, or until the onion appears translucent and the peppers and cauliflower have softened. Continue to add water if needed to prevent sticking.

4. Add the garlic, and cook, stirring, for 1 minute, or until fragrant.

5. Season with the salt, pepper, and turmeric. Stir gently for 2 to 3 minutes, or until heated through. Remove from the heat.

Per Serving: Calories: 111; Total fat: 5g; Saturated fat: 1g; Protein: 3g; Total carbohydrates: 15g; Fiber: 4g; Sugar: 5g; Cholesterol: 0g

→ **VARIATION:** Consider adding mushrooms or spinach (or both) with the seasonings in step 5. Cook for 2 to 4 minutes, or until soft.

Mushroom and Tofu Scramble

Dairy-Free, Gluten-Free, Nut-Free, Vegan

SERVES 4

PREP TIME: 5 MINUTES / COOK TIME: 10 MINUTES

Tofu scrambles as well as eggs and is a great vegan-friendly protein option that has both antiangiogenic and DNA health properties. It also contains antioxidants and calcium. It pairs well with all vegetables, but especially savory mushrooms. Consider serving this scramble with a slice of sourdough toast and some balsamic vinegar–dressed greens.

2 tablespoons extra-virgin olive oil

½ yellow onion, diced

2 garlic cloves, minced

8 ounces (2 cups) sliced mushrooms

1 (12-ounce) package firm tofu, pressed and crumbled

1 teaspoon turmeric

¾ teaspoon salt

½ teaspoon freshly ground black pepper

Bioactive ingredients: onion, garlic, mushroom, tofu, turmeric

1. In a large skillet, heat the oil over medium heat.

2. Add the onion, and sauté for 3 to 5 minutes, or until translucent.

3. Add the garlic and mushrooms. Cook for 2 to 3 minutes, or until the mushrooms have softened and the garlic is fragrant.

4. Add the tofu, and sauté for 4 to 5 minutes, or until slightly browned. If the tofu sticks to the skillet, add 1 teaspoon of water, and lightly scrape the bottom.

5. Stir in the turmeric, salt, and pepper. Remove from the heat. Serve hot.

Per Serving: Calories: 206; Total fat: 14g; Saturated fat: 2g; Protein: 15g; Total carbohydrates: 8g; Fiber: 3g; Sugar: 2g; Cholesterol: 0g

→ **VARIATION:** You can use any type of vegetables you like as a replacement for the mushrooms in this scramble. Some options include peppers, tomato, scallions, broccoli or broccoli rabe, or zucchini. Depending on what you use, you may need to increase the cooking time. You can also add some shredded cheese if you like; consider Gouda or muenster.

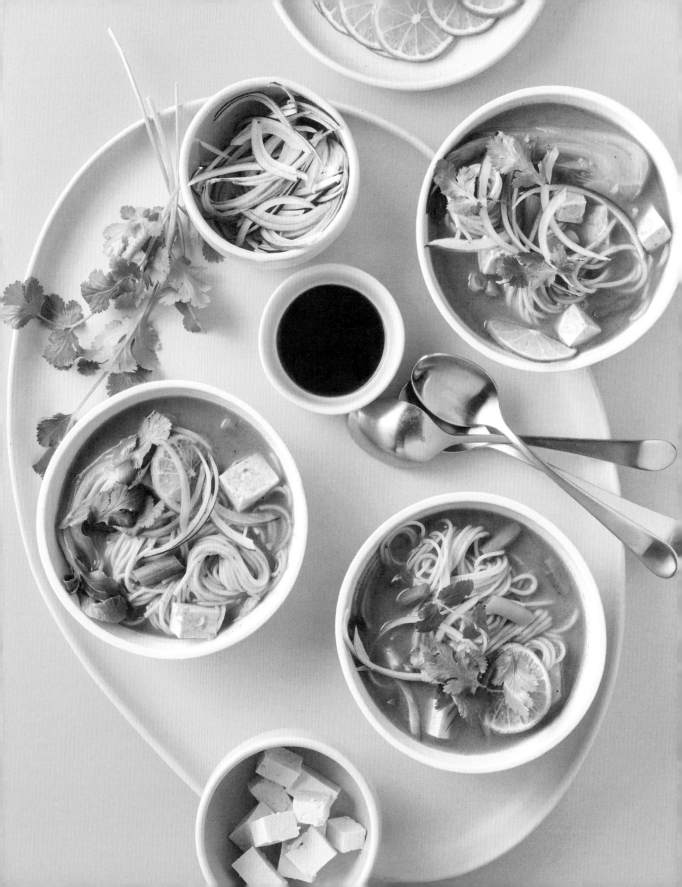

CHAPTER 4

Salads and Soups

By stocking your kitchen with simple yet health-promoting ingredients, you will be ready to whip up soups and salads for lunch or dinner that boost your natural defense systems. Whatever your cooking skills and time available to prepare meals, there are options in this chapter for you. Many are no-cook and use pantry items like canned beans, root vegetables, and dry goods, such as oats and nuts. The majority of these recipes are plant based, with some chicken and seafood options as well.

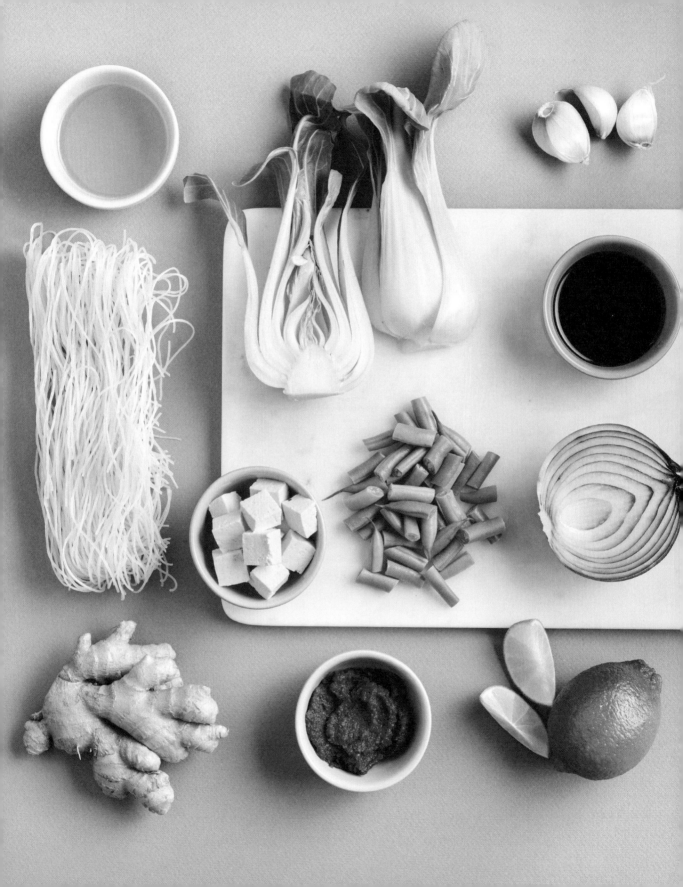

Easy Curry Noodle Soup

Dairy-Free, Nut-Free, Vegan

SERVES 4

PREP TIME: 5 MINUTES / COOK TIME: 20 MINUTES

Not only is this soup comforting and savory, but also it provides a unique array of health benefits that support the five defense systems. The best part is that it is quick and easy to prepare. You simply sauté the vegetables, spices, and tofu, then add the liquid and pour the hot soup over the noodles.

2½ tablespoons extra-virgin olive oil

1 cup chopped green beans

2 heads baby bok choy, quartered

3 garlic cloves, minced

2 tablespoons grated fresh ginger

¼ cup Thai red curry paste

1 (12-ounce) package firm tofu, pressed and diced

5 cups vegetable stock

2½ tablespoons low-sodium soy sauce

⅔ cup light coconut milk

8 ounces dried rice vermicelli noodles

1 lime, cut into wedges

½ red onion, thinly sliced

Bioactive ingredients: olive oil, green bean, bok choy, garlic, ginger, tofu, soy sauce, onion

1. In a large stockpot, heat the oil over medium heat.

2. Add the green beans and bok choy. Sauté for 5 minutes, or until starting to soften.

3. Add the garlic, ginger, and curry paste. Cook, stirring, for 2 minutes, or until fragrant.

4. Add the tofu, stirring very gently so it doesn't crumble, and cook for 4 to 6 minutes, or until lightly browned. Add water, 1 tablespoon at a time, if needed to prevent excessive sticking to the pot.

5. Add the stock, soy sauce, and coconut milk. Bring to a boil. Remove from the heat.

6. Divide the noodles among 4 serving bowls.

7. Pour the hot soup over the noodles in 4 equal amounts. Let sit for 2 to 4 minutes to allow the noodles to soften completely.

8. Top each soup bowl with a slice of lime and a quarter of the red onion.

Per Serving: Calories: 465; Total fat: 19g; Saturated fat: 3g; Protein: 20g; Total carbohydrates: 59g; Fiber: 6g; Sugar: 2g; Cholesterol: 0g

Spicy Black Bean and Coconut Soup

Dairy-Free, Gluten-Free,
Nut-Free, Soy-Free, Vegan

SERVES 6

PREP TIME: 10 MINUTES / COOK TIME: 30 MINUTES

This protein-packed soup is full of fiber and flavor. *Eat to Beat Disease* generally recommends a lower saturated fat intake, so I use light coconut milk. Feel free to use full-fat coconut milk if you prefer. You can easily reduce or eliminate the spices in this recipe for a milder soup.

2 tablespoons coconut oil

½ yellow onion, diced

3 garlic cloves, minced

2½ cups water

1 (14-ounce) can light coconut milk

1 jalapeño, diced

¼ teaspoon ground allspice

2 teaspoons ground cumin

½ teaspoon chili powder

1 teaspoon salt

3 (15½-ounce) cans black beans, drained and rinsed

Juice of 1 medium lime

¼ cup unsweetened shredded coconut flakes

¼ cup chopped fresh cilantro

Bioactive ingredients: onion, garlic, chile, cumin, beans

1. In a large stockpot, heat the oil over medium-high heat.

2. Add the onion, and cook, stirring often, for 2 to 3 minutes, or until translucent.

3. Add the garlic, and cook for 1 minute, or until fragrant.

4. Add the water, coconut milk, jalapeño, allspice, cumin, chili powder, and salt. Bring to a simmer.

5. Add the beans. Cook, stirring occasionally, for 20 minutes, or until the flavors meld. Remove from the heat.

6. Using an immersion blender, blend about a quarter of the soup until smooth, leaving most of the beans whole for texture.

7. Mix in the lime juice.

8. Garnish with the coconut flakes and cilantro.

Per Serving: Calories: 385; Total fat: 22g; Saturated fat: 19g; Protein: 13g; Total carbohydrates: 37g; Fiber: 13g; Sugar: 3g; Cholesterol: 0g

→ **VARIATION:** If you don't like spice, you can swap out the jalapeño for a milder version like an Anaheim pepper. You could also make this soup with a different type of bean, such as navy or white.

Savory Vegetarian Navy Bean Soup

Dairy-Free, Gluten-Free, Nut-Free, Soy-Free, Vegan, Vegetarian

SERVES 6

PREP TIME: 10 MINUTES / COOK TIME: 1 HOUR 10 MINUTES

Most navy bean soup recipes include some sort of ham or pork product, which creates a savory, salty flavor that complements the beans. But there are other ways to make a warm and comforting navy bean soup, like using savory vegetable stock, root vegetables, and herbs and spices to create a rich-tasting, plant-based soup.

1 tablespoon extra-virgin olive oil

1 large yellow onion, diced

3 carrots, cut into thin rounds

3 celery stalks, diced

1 red bell pepper, seeded and diced

4 garlic cloves, minced

4 (15½-ounce) cans white beans, rinsed and drained

1 tablespoon fresh thyme leaves

1 tablespoon plus 1 teaspoon ground cumin

1 teaspoon salt

½ teaspoon freshly ground black pepper

8 cups vegetable stock

¼ cup chopped fresh parsley

Bioactive ingredients: olive oil, onion, carrot, celery, bell pepper, garlic, beans, thyme, cumin, parsley

1. In a large stockpot, heat the oil over medium heat.

2. Add the onion, carrots, celery, bell pepper, and garlic. Sauté for 4 to 6 minutes, or until softened.

3. Add the beans, thyme, cumin, salt, pepper, and stock. Bring to a boil.

4. Reduce the heat to low. Cover the pot, and simmer, stirring occasionally, for 1 hour, or until the vegetables are very soft. Remove from the heat.

5. Transfer 2 cups of the soup to a blender. Blend until smooth, then return to the pot (or use an immersion blender in the pot to puree about a quarter of the soup). This will give the soup a thicker, creamier texture.

6. Stir in the parsley. Serve hot.

Per Serving: Calories: 292; Total fat: 3g; Saturated fat: 1g; Protein: 18g; Total carbohydrates: 50g; Fiber: 13g; Sugar: 3g; Cholesterol: 0g

Roasted Root Vegetable Soup

Dairy-Free, Gluten-Free,
Nut-Free, Soy-Free, Vegan

SERVES 6

PREP TIME: 30 MINUTES / COOK TIME: 50 MINUTES

Even though roasted root vegetables may remind you of a cozy dish for cold weather, this is a perfect soup to make all year round. Root vegetables last for a long time in the pantry, so this is a great way to make a meal with vegetables you already have on hand.

2 medium parsnips, peeled and diced

1 medium rutabaga, peeled and diced

2 medium turnips, peeled and diced

2 medium carrots, peeled and diced

1 medium sweet potato, peeled and diced

4 teaspoons extra-virgin olive oil, divided

1¼ teaspoons salt, divided

½ teaspoon freshly ground black pepper, divided

½ yellow onion, diced

2 garlic cloves, minced

1½ teaspoons fresh thyme leaves

1 teaspoon fresh rosemary leaves, chopped

8 cups vegetable stock

1. Preheat the oven to 450°F.

2. Distribute the parsnips, rutabaga, turnips, carrots, and sweet potato evenly over 2 large sheet pans.

3. Drizzle each sheet with 1½ teaspoons of oil. Season each with ½ teaspoon of salt and ¼ teaspoon of pepper.

4. Transfer the sheet pans to the oven, and roast for 15 minutes. Flip the vegetables so they cook evenly, and roast for 15 minutes, or until softened. Remove from the oven.

5. In a large stockpot, heat the remaining 1 teaspoon of oil over medium heat.

6. Add the onion, and cook for 2 to 3 minutes, or until translucent.

7. Add the garlic, thyme, rosemary, and remaining ¼ teaspoon of salt. Cook, stirring frequently, for 1 minute.

8. Add the roasted vegetables and stock. Bring to a boil.

9. Reduce the heat to low. Simmer for 10 minutes, or until the vegetables are soft enough to pierce using a fork. Remove from the heat.

Per Serving: Calories: 127; Total fat: 3g; Saturated fat: 0g; Protein: 2g; Total carbohydrates: 24g; Fiber: 6g; Sugar: 9g; Cholesterol: 0g

→ **VARIATION:** For additional nutritional and health benefits, garnish each dish with 1 teaspoon fresh or dried thyme, rosemary, or parsley leaves, or a combination.

Bioactive ingredients: rutabaga, turnip, carrot, sweet potato, olive oil, onion, garlic, thyme, rosemary

Simple Greens with Apple Cider Vinegar Dressing

Dairy-Free, Gluten-Free, Nut-Free, Soy-Free, Vegetarian

SERVES 4 (½ CUP DRESSING)

PREP TIME: 10 MINUTES

Making your own dressing gives you flavor minus the preservatives, stabilizers, and additives often found in shelf-stable varieties. You can whip up a dressing in minutes in a Mason jar with a lid and keep it in your refrigerator. Simply give it a shake just before serving, and you can enjoy this salad all week long.

¼ cup extra-virgin olive oil

2 tablespoons apple cider vinegar

2 teaspoons honey

½ teaspoon Dijon mustard

1 garlic clove, minced

1 teaspoon chopped dried rosemary

¼ teaspoon salt

⅛ teaspoon freshly ground black pepper

1 head red-leaf lettuce, chopped or torn into bite-size pieces

Bioactive ingredients: olive oil, garlic, rosemary, red-leaf lettuce

1. To make the dressing, in a medium mixing bowl, whisk together the oil, vinegar, honey, mustard, garlic, rosemary, salt, and pepper.

2. Divide the lettuce evenly among 4 bowls.

3. Drizzle each bowl with a quarter of the dressing.

Per Serving: Calories: 146; Total fat: 14g; Saturated fat: 2g; Protein: 1g; Total carbohydrates: 5g; Fiber: 1g; Sugar: 3g; Cholesterol: 0g

→ **VARIATION:** The dressing will keep for 5 days when stored in an airtight container in the refrigerator, so consider making a double or triple batch for the week as needed. You can mix up the herbs and spices for different flavors: consider ¼ teaspoon chili powder, cayenne, or paprika for a little kick and even more anti-oxidants. Instead of or in addition to lettuce, consider using kale, spinach, or arugula.

Tomato-Basil White Bean and Quinoa Salad

Dairy-Free, Gluten-Free, Nut-Free, Soy-Free, Vegan

SERVES 5

PREP TIME: 10 MINUTES / COOK TIME: 25 MINUTES

If you need a year-round salad that you can make ahead at home or take to parties or picnics, this is it. Perfectly balanced with whole-grain quinoa and protein-rich beans, this hearty salad gets a bright pop of flavor from fresh herbs and produce that add health benefits, too.

¾ cup quinoa, rinsed

1½ cups water

1 (15-ounce) can white beans, drained and rinsed

¼ cup diced red onion

1 cup cherry tomatoes, halved

3 tablespoons chopped fresh basil leaves

2 tablespoons extra-virgin olive oil

1 tablespoon red wine vinegar

1 teaspoon freshly squeezed lemon juice

¼ teaspoon salt

¼ teaspoon freshly ground black pepper

Bioactive ingredients: quinoa, beans, onion, tomato, basil, olive oil, lemon

1. In a medium saucepan, combine the quinoa and water. Bring to a boil over medium-high heat.

2. Reduce the heat to low. Cover the saucepan, and simmer for 15 minutes, or until all the water has been absorbed. Remove from the heat. Let sit, covered, for 5 minutes. Using a fork, fluff the cooked quinoa. Let cool for about 10 minutes, or until just warm, not hot.

3. Meanwhile, put the beans, onion, tomatoes, and basil in a large mixing bowl.

4. In a small mixing bowl, whisk together the oil, vinegar, lemon juice, salt, and pepper.

5. Add the warm quinoa to the large bowl. Mix gently to combine.

6. Drizzle the dressing over the quinoa mixture, and stir gently until the ingredients are coated.

Per Serving: Calories: 226; Total fat: 7g; Saturated fat: 1g; Protein: 9g; Total carbohydrates: 32g; Fiber: 6g; Sugar: 1g; Cholesterol: 0g

→ **VARIATION:** Consider adding some Parmigiano-Reggiano as a garnish for additional flavor and microbiome support.

Creamy Purple Potato Salad

Gluten-Free, Nut-Free,
Soy-Free, Vegetarian

SERVES 4

PREP TIME: 10 MINUTES / COOK TIME:
20 MINUTES, PLUS 10 MINUTES TO COOL

Classic potato salad gets a healthy boost in this version that swaps out white potatoes for higher-antioxidant purple potatoes. This easy salad features microbiome-supporting yogurt rather than mayonnaise and plenty of dried and fresh herbs for flavor and health benefits.

2 pounds small purple potatoes, quartered

2 ears of corn, shucked and kernels removed

1 cup nonfat plain Greek yogurt or nondairy yogurt

1 teaspoon Dijon mustard

2 garlic cloves, minced

1 teaspoon freshly squeezed lemon juice

½ teaspoon dried basil

½ teaspoon dried oregano

¼ teaspoon dried dill

¼ cup chopped fresh parsley

1 teaspoon salt

½ teaspoon freshly ground black pepper

Bioactive ingredients: purple potato, yogurt, garlic, lemon, basil, oregano, parsley

1. Put the potatoes in a large stockpot, and cover with water by 2 to 3 inches. Bring to a boil over high heat.

2. Reduce the heat to medium. Boil the potatoes for 12 to 15 minutes, or until easily pierced with a fork.

3. Add the corn during the last 2 minutes of cooking time. Remove from the heat. Drain. Let cool for 5 to 10 minutes.

4. Meanwhile, in a large mixing bowl, whisk together the yogurt, mustard, garlic, lemon juice, basil, oregano, dill, parsley, salt, and pepper.

5. Add the cooled potatoes and corn. Stir gently to coat.

Per Serving: Calories: 261; Total fat: 1g; Saturated fat: 0g; Protein: 11g; Total carbohydrates: 53g; Fiber: 7g; Sugar: 7g; Cholesterol: 4g

→ **VARIATION:** If you don't have access to fresh corn on the cob, because it's out of season or it isn't available where you live, feel free to use 2 cups frozen kernels, and add them to the boiling water for 1 minute. If you can't find purple potatoes, feel free to use baby red potatoes instead.

Chickpea and Avocado Salad

Dairy-Free, Gluten-Free,
Nut-Free, Soy-Free, Vegan

SERVES 4

PREP TIME: 10 MINUTES

A hearty salad perfect for lunch or a snack, this recipe can be made in minutes and requires no cooking. Because it's not lettuce based, it is ideal for making ahead and storing in the refrigerator, so you always have a health-boosting, filling meal option on hand.

2 (15-ounce) cans chickpeas, drained and rinsed

½ small red onion, diced

2 garlic cloves, minced

Grated zest of 1 lime

Juice of 4 limes

½ cup chopped fresh cilantro

2 tablespoons chopped scallions, green and white parts

¾ teaspoon salt

1 ripe avocado, halved, pitted, peeled, and diced

Bioactive ingredients: beans, onion, garlic, avocado

1. In a medium mixing bowl, combine the chickpeas, onion, garlic, lime zest, lime juice, cilantro, scallions, and salt. Mix well.

2. Just before serving, fold the avocado gently into the salad. Store covered in an airtight container in the refrigerator for up to 4 days.

Per Serving: Calories: 267; Total fat: 11g; Saturated fat: 2g; Protein: 10g; Total carbohydrates: 37g; Fiber: 12g; Sugar: 8g; Cholesterol: 0g

→ **VARIATION:** You could make this salad with other types of beans, though chickpeas are ideal because of their firm texture. Feel free to use spices, like ¼ teaspoon cayenne or chili powder, or even add a diced jalapeño for spicier flavor.

Kale Caesar with Parmigiano-Reggiano and Homemade Croutons

Nut-Free, Soy-Free

SERVES 6

PREP TIME: 15 MINUTES / COOK TIME: 10 MINUTES

Hearty (and healthy!) kale leaves become much softer when they're incorporated into a salad with the right dressing. Chop the leaves small so that the dressing coats them fully. This is a perfect side dish, or it can stand alone as a healthy lunch or dinner if you add a protein source like beans, tofu, tempeh, chicken, or salmon. Feel free to make the croutons from store-bought or homemade sourdough (page 140).

4 cups diced (1-inch) rustic sourdough bread

¼ cup extra-virgin olive oil

2 garlic cloves, minced

¾ teaspoon salt, divided

½ teaspoon freshly ground black pepper, divided

¼ cup tahini

½ teaspoon Dijon mustard

1½ tablespoons freshly squeezed lemon juice

1½ teaspoons white wine vinegar

⅓ cup grated Parmigiano-Reggiano cheese, plus 2 tablespoons

6 cups hand-torn kale leaves (bite-size pieces)

1 large head red-leaf lettuce, chopped into bite-size pieces

1. Preheat the oven to 400°F.

2. Spread the bread out in a single layer on a sheet pan.

3. Transfer the sheet pan to the oven, and bake for 8 to 10 minutes, or until the croutons are golden brown. Remove from the oven.

4. Meanwhile, in a large mixing bowl, combine the oil, garlic, ½ teaspoon of salt, and ¼ teaspoon of pepper.

5. To make the dressing, in a blender or food processor, combine the tahini, mustard, lemon juice, vinegar, remaining ¼ teaspoon of salt and ¼ teaspoon of pepper, and ⅓ cup of cheese. Puree for about 30 seconds, or until smooth.

6. Add the croutons to the large bowl, and toss to coat evenly.

7. In another large bowl, combine the kale and lettuce.

8. Drizzle the dressing over the top of the greens, and using your hands, lightly massage the dressing into the greens until well dressed.

9. Add the croutons and remaining 2 tablespoons of cheese.

Per Serving: Calories: 238; Total fat: 17g; Saturated fat: 3g; Protein: 6g; Total carbohydrates: 17g; Fiber: 3g; Sugar: 2g; Cholesterol: 5g

→ **VARIATION:** You can use different types of greens with this salad. Kale offers a nice, hearty texture, but you can also use romaine, arugula, spinach, or even chopped collard greens in your salad mix.

Bioactive ingredients: sourdough bread, olive oil, garlic, tahini, lemon, Parmigiano-Reggiano, kale, red-leaf lettuce

Eggplant Salad with Walnuts and Mint

Dairy-Free, Gluten-Free, Soy-Free, Vegetarian

SERVES 4

PREP TIME: 5 MINUTES / COOK TIME: 40 MINUTES

This simple warm salad comes together quickly, making it a perfect weeknight meal for the family, yet elegant enough for guests. It's an unexpected side dish that's full of health-promoting vegetables, nuts, and herbs.

¾ cup walnuts

2 tablespoons freshly squeezed lemon juice

1 tablespoon honey

½ teaspoon ground cinnamon

½ teaspoon salt

4 tablespoons extra-virgin olive oil, divided

1 large eggplant, cut into 1-inch dice

¼ cup chopped fresh mint leaves

Bioactive ingredients: walnut, lemon, cinnamon, olive oil, eggplant, mint

1. Preheat the oven to 350°F.

2. Spread the walnuts out on a sheet pan. Transfer the sheet pan to the oven, and toast for 4 to 5 minutes. Flip the walnuts, and toast for another 4 to 5 minutes, or until golden brown and fragrant. Remove from the oven, leaving the oven on.

3. Increase the oven temperature to 400°F.

4. Meanwhile, in a large bowl, whisk together the lemon juice, honey, cinnamon, and salt. Whisk in 1 tablespoon of oil.

5. Put the eggplant on a sheet pan. Drizzle with the remaining 3 tablespoons of oil. Transfer the sheet pan to the oven, and bake for 15 minutes. Flip the eggplant, and bake for 15 minutes, or until golden brown. Remove from the oven.

6. While the eggplant is baking, coarsely chop the walnuts.

7. Add the eggplant while still warm to the bowl, and gently toss to combine.

8. Garnish with the mint and walnuts. Serve warm.

Per Serving: Calories: 316; Total fat: 28g; Saturated fat: 3g; Protein: 5g; Total carbohydrates: 16g; Fiber: 6g; Sugar: 10g; Cholesterol: 0g

Creamy Mushroom Soup

Dairy-Free, Gluten-Free,
Nut-Free, Vegan

SERVES 5

PREP TIME: 10 MINUTES / COOK TIME: 20 TO
25 MINUTES, PLUS 10 MINUTES TO COOL

This soup has a secret: it's completely dairy-free but has the texture and substance of a cream-based soup, thanks to the oats that are cooked in the broth and then pureed together with the other ingredients. When the soup has cooled, finish it with miso so as not to destroy the good bacteria in the miso that can help support gut health with high heat.

1 tablespoon extra-virgin olive oil

1 large yellow onion, chopped

3 garlic cloves, minced

1 teaspoon salt

½ teaspoon freshly ground black pepper

1 teaspoon dried oregano

1 pound mushrooms, chopped (3 to 4 cups)

4 cups vegetable stock

1½ cups water

⅔ cup rolled oats

2 tablespoons miso

Bioactive ingredients: olive oil, onion, garlic, oregano, mushroom, oats, miso

1. In a large stockpot, heat the oil over medium heat.

2. Add the onion, and sauté for 5 to 6 minutes, or until translucent.

3. Add the garlic, salt, pepper, oregano, and mushrooms. Cook for 1 minute, adding 1 tablespoon of water if needed to prevent sticking.

4. Add the stock, water, and oats. Bring to a boil.

5. Reduce the heat to medium. Cover the pot, and cook for 8 to 10 minutes, or until the oats are soft. Remove from the heat. Remove the lid, and let cool for 5 to 10 minutes.

6. Using an immersion blender or in batches in a blender with a tight-fitting lid, puree the soup until smooth.

7. Add the miso, and stir until completely incorporated.

Per Serving: Calories: 139; Total fat: 5g; Saturated fat: 1g; Protein: 7g; Total carbohydrates: 20g; Fiber: 4g; Sugar: 4g; Cholesterol: 0g

Stone Fruit Salad with Honey Vinaigrette

Dairy-Free, Gluten-Free,
Soy-Free, Vegetarian

SERVES 4

PREP TIME: 10 MINUTES

Brighten up your next fruit salad by choosing stone fruit like cherries, plums, peaches, and nectarines, which are rich in vitamins, minerals, and disease-fighting antioxidants. This type of fruit holds up well if you chop it ahead of time to mix with the greens and dressing for a quick meal or snack during the week.

2 tablespoons extra-virgin olive oil

1 tablespoon apple cider vinegar

1 tablespoon honey

½ teaspoon ground cinnamon

2 teaspoons chopped fresh mint leaves

2 apricots, pitted and sliced

1 nectarine, pitted and sliced

1 plum, pitted and sliced

1 cup cherries, pitted and halved

3 cups spinach

3 cups arugula

½ cup sliced almonds

Bioactive ingredients: olive oil, cinnamon, mint, apricot, nectarine, plum, cherry, spinach, arugula, almond

1. To make the vinaigrette, in a small mixing bowl or in a Mason jar with a lid, combine the oil, vinegar, honey, cinnamon, and mint. Whisk together, or shake in the jar.

2. In a medium mixing bowl, stir together the apricots, nectarine, plum, and cherries.

3. In a large mixing bowl, combine the spinach and arugula.

4. Drizzle with half of the vinaigrette, and toss to coat.

5. Pour the stone fruit on top of the greens, and drizzle with the remaining vinaigrette.

6. Garnish with the almonds.

Per Serving: Calories: 209; Total fat: 13g; Saturated fat: 1g; Protein: 5g; Total carbohydrates: 22g; Fiber: 4g; Sugar: 16g; Cholesterol: 0g

→ **VARIATION:** If you don't have access to fresh, ripe stone fruit or it's out of season, consider using frozen, canned, or dried varieties instead.

5-Minute Salmon Salad

Gluten-Free, Nut-Free, Soy-Free

SERVES 4

PREP TIME: 5 MINUTES

For a protein-packed salad that you can make in minutes and that requires hardly any preparation at all, use canned salmon and some simple vegetables and herbs. Serve it on a sandwich or crackers, or try it over greens for lunch. Alternatively, package it for use later in the week for a grab-and-go lunch or snack.

2 (5-ounce) cans salmon, drained

¼ cup nonfat plain Greek yogurt or soy yogurt

1 medium celery stalk, diced

½ small to medium cucumber, diced

3 tablespoons finely chopped scallions, green and white parts

1 tablespoon chopped fresh dill

¼ teaspoon salt

¼ teaspoon freshly ground black pepper

1 tablespoon freshly squeezed lemon juice

Bioactive ingredients: salmon, yogurt, celery, onion, lemon

In a small mixing bowl, combine the salmon, yogurt, celery, cucumber, scallions, dill, salt, pepper, and lemon juice. Mix well. Store covered in the refrigerator for up to 4 days.

Per Serving: Calories: 111; Total fat: 4g; Saturated fat: 1g; Protein: 16g; Total carbohydrates: 3g; Fiber: 1g; Sugar: 1g; Cholesterol: 39g

→ **VARIATION:** Consider using an equal portion of canned tuna instead of salmon. Swap in or out any vegetables that you prefer. One medium carrot, ½ bell pepper, or both work well and add even more health benefits.

Mediterranean-Style Tuna Salad with Olives

Dairy-Free, Gluten-Free, Nut-Free, Soy-Free

SERVES 4

PREP TIME: 10 MINUTES

Tuna salad is another quick, versatile option and makes for a perfect snack or light meal. The fermented vegetables—olives and capers—add gut health support for a strong microbiome.

2 teaspoons Dijon mustard

Grated zest and juice of 1 lemon

2 tablespoons extra-virgin olive oil

½ teaspoon dried oregano

½ teaspoon dried basil

¼ teaspoon salt

⅛ teaspoon freshly ground black pepper

2 (5-ounce) cans tuna, drained

2 celery stalks, diced

4 small radishes, chopped

½ red onion, finely chopped

½ cup Kalamata olives, pitted and halved

3 tablespoons chopped fresh parsley

3 tablespoons chopped fresh dill

2 tablespoons capers

Bioactive ingredients: lemon, olive oil, oregano, basil, tuna, celery, onion, parsley, capers

1. To make the dressing, in a small mixing bowl, whisk together the mustard, lemon zest and juice, oil, oregano, basil, salt, and pepper.

2. In a large mixing bowl, gently mix together the tuna, celery, radishes, onion, olives, parsley, and dill.

3. Pour the dressing over the tuna salad, and mix until the vegetables are coated.

4. Garnish with the capers, and serve chilled.

Per Serving: Calories: 159; Total fat: 10g; Saturated fat: 1g; Protein: 13g; Total carbohydrates: 7g; Fiber: 3g; Sugar: 1g; Cholesterol: 20g

→ **VARIATION:** Adjust the herbs and spices in this recipe to fit your taste; consider fresh oregano or basil in the dressing. You could also swap out the lemon zest and juice for lime for a slightly different flavor. Adding red pepper flakes adds a nice kick if you like some heat.

Waldorf Chicken Salad

Gluten-Free, Soy-Free

SERVES 4

PREP TIME: 10 MINUTES

Celebrate a perfect combination of fruits, vegetables, nuts, and chicken in this new twist on a classic salad. Greek yogurt adds tanginess and microbiome-boosting benefits as well as protein and calcium. This is a great way to use up leftover chicken from a rotisserie or roast earlier in the week.

½ cup nonfat plain Greek yogurt or soy yogurt

3 tablespoons apple cider vinegar

1 tablespoon honey

2 tablespoons chopped fresh parsley

½ teaspoon salt

¼ teaspoon freshly ground black pepper

2 cups chopped cooked chicken leg or thigh meat

2 celery stalks, diced

1 Granny Smith apple, cored and diced

1 cup seedless red grapes, halved

¾ cup pecans, chopped

4 cups chopped red-leaf lettuce

2 tablespoons chopped chives

Bioactive ingredients: yogurt, parsley, chicken, celery, apple, grape, pecan, red-leaf lettuce

1. To make the dressing, in a small mixing bowl, whisk together the yogurt, vinegar, honey, parsley, salt, and pepper.

2. In a large mixing bowl, gently combine the chicken, celery, apple, grapes, and pecans.

3. Add the dressing, and mix gently to incorporate.

4. Divide the lettuce evenly among 4 serving bowls.

5. Top each serving with a quarter of the chicken salad.

6. Garnish with the chives.

Per Serving: Calories: 345; Total fat: 20g; Saturated fat: 2g; Protein: 21g; Total carbohydrates: 22g; Fiber: 4g; Sugar: 17g; Cholesterol: 56g

→ **VARIATION:** Consider using the same quantity of canned chicken for an even faster prep time if you don't have cooked chicken on hand. Or simply eliminate the chicken for a vegetarian option. You can swap out the apple for the same amount of chopped pear and use any color of grapes that you prefer.

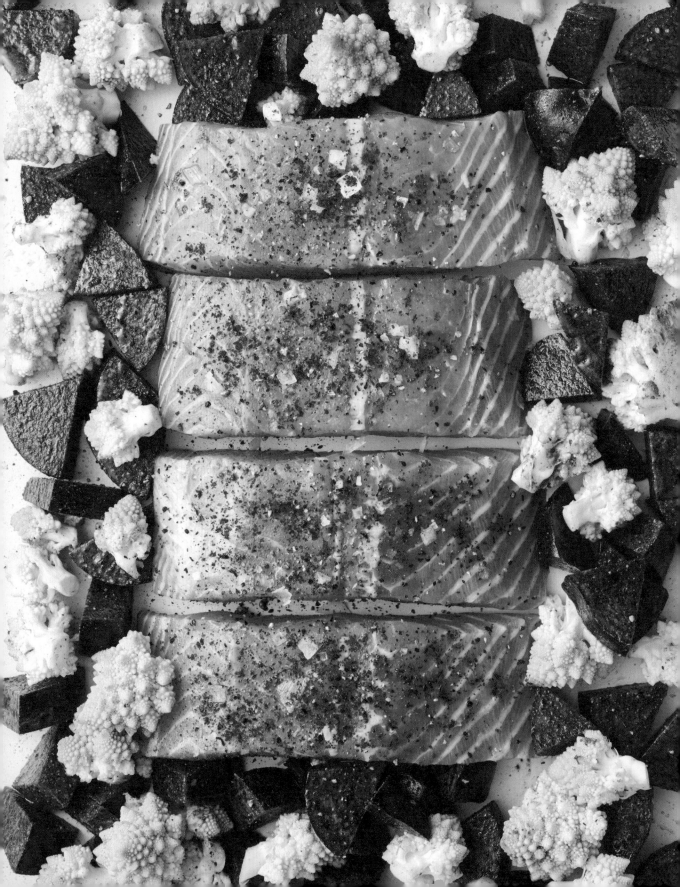

CHAPTER 5

Seafood

Fish and shellfish take center stage when it comes to antiangiogenic omega-3 fatty acids in the diet. Omega-3s also get a lot of attention as a healthy fat that supports the cardiovascular system. The types of fish highest in omega-3 fatty acids include clams, some types of tuna, salmon, halibut, herring, mackerel, arctic char, sardines, swordfish, squid, and rainbow trout. When choosing seafood, there's more to consider than what's good for your individual health; there's also the health of the oceans and our environment. The fish in this chapter are those that come from sustainable sources. Notably, aquaculture has come a long way, and some farmed seafood is actually among the highest in quality and environmental sustainability. Choose your seafood carefully, and experiment with the most sustainable varieties, such as farmed arctic char, mussels, clams, and trout.

69

Lemon-Garlic Steamed Clams

Gluten-Free, Nut-Free,
Soy-Free

SERVES 4

PREP TIME: 5 MINUTES / COOK TIME: 20 MINUTES

A bowl of savory garlic steamed clams accompanied by fresh, crusty sour-dough bread (see page 140) is a perfect comfort food. There are some really exciting changes in aquaculture, especially around farmed clams and mussels, so don't hesitate to purchase clams that are farmed; it could be a great choice for you—and the environment.

3 tablespoons
    butter, divided

3 garlic cloves, minced

¼ cup chopped shallot

1½ cups dry white wine

1½ cups vegetable stock

3 pounds small clams, rinsed
    and scrubbed

¼ cup coconut cream
    (from the top of a can of
    coconut milk)

Juice of ½ lemon

½ lemon, thinly sliced

½ cup chopped fresh parsley

Bioactive ingredients: garlic,
white wine, clams, lemon,
parsley

1. In a large skillet, melt 2 tablespoons of butter over medium heat.

2. Add the garlic and shallot. Cook, stirring occasionally, for 2 to 4 minutes, or until starting to soften.

3. Add the wine and stock. Bring to a boil.

4. Reduce the heat to medium to achieve a rolling simmer. Add the clams, cover the skillet, and cook for 6 to 8 minutes, or until the clams have opened up. Remove from the heat.

5. Stir in the coconut cream, lemon juice, and remaining 1 tablespoon of butter. Discard any clams that haven't opened.

6. Garnish with the lemon slices and parsley.

Per Serving: Calories: 238; Total fat: 12g; Saturated fat: 8g; Protein: 9g; Total carbohydrates: 8g; Fiber: 1g; Sugar: 2g; Cholesterol: 38g

→ **VARIATION:** You can easily substitute mussels for the clams, but make sure to debeard them before cooking (remove any fibers from the shell) and then increase the cook time to 10 to 15 minutes, or until the mussels open up.

Quick Tuna Patties

Dairy-Free, Nut-Free,
Soy-Free

SERVES 4

PREP TIME: 10 MINUTES / COOK TIME: 10 MINUTES

A quick and easy lunch or dinner, homemade tuna patties are a delicious source of protein and healthy fats. Tuna patties resemble a crab cake because you use bread crumbs and egg as a binder. However, tuna is higher in omega-3 fatty acids and is not only versatile but also affordable. Consider serving these as an appetizer over greens like arugula or spinach.

2 (5-ounce) cans
  tuna, drained

2 teaspoons Dijon mustard

½ cup small hand-torn
  pieces sourdough bread

2 tablespoons freshly
  squeezed lemon juice

1 teaspoon grated
  lemon zest

2 tablespoons chopped
  fresh parsley

2 tablespoons chopped
  scallions, light green and
  white parts

1 celery stalk, chopped

½ teaspoon salt

½ teaspoon freshly ground
  black pepper

1 egg

2 tablespoons extra-virgin
  olive oil

Bioactive ingredients: tuna,
sourdough bread, lemon,
parsley, onion, celery,
olive oil

1. Line a sheet pan with wax paper.

2. In a medium mixing bowl, combine the tuna, mustard, bread, lemon juice, lemon zest, parsley, scallions, celery, salt, pepper, and egg. Mix well.

3. Divide the tuna mixture into 4 equal parts on the prepared sheet pan.

4. Using your hands, shape each serving into a ball, then gently flatten each into a patty.

5. In a large skillet, heat the oil over medium-high heat.

6. Add the patties, and cook for about 4 minutes per side, or until golden brown. Remove from the heat.

Per Serving: Calories: 144; Total fat: 9g; Saturated fat: 1g; Protein: 13g; Total carbohydrates: 4g; Fiber: 1g; Sugar: 1g; Cholesterol: 67g

→ **VARIATION:** Consider using canned salmon or crab for variety. You could use ½ cup panko bread crumbs instead of the sourdough if it is more convenient.

Classic Cioppino

Dairy-Free, Gluten-Free, Nut-Free, Soy-Free	**SERVES 4** PREP TIME: 15 MINUTES / COOK TIME: 35 TO 40 MINUTES

A classic, stock-based seafood stew, cioppino is a simple, one-pot way to combine high-omega-3 fish and shellfish. Popular in my native Pacific Northwest, cioppino is made especially in areas that have access to a variety of fish and shellfish options. Be sure to serve it with some fresh sourdough bread (see page 140).

1½ tablespoons extra-virgin olive oil

1 medium yellow onion, diced

½ fennel bulb, thinly sliced

1 celery stalk, chopped

1 large carrot, peeled and chopped

2 garlic cloves, minced

1 teaspoon salt

½ teaspoon freshly ground black pepper

½ teaspoon red pepper flakes

2 tablespoons tomato paste

1 large tomato, diced

¾ cup dry white wine

3 cups vegetable stock

8 ounces clams, scrubbed

8 ounces mussels, scrubbed and debearded

8 ounces salmon, skin removed, cut into 2-inch dice

¼ cup chopped fresh parsley

½ lemon, thinly sliced

Bioactive ingredients: olive oil, onion, celery, carrot, garlic, tomato, white wine, clams, salmon, parsley, lemon

1. In a large pot, heat the oil over medium heat.

2. Add the onion and fennel. Sauté, stirring, for 3 minutes, or until fragrant.

3. Add the celery, carrot, and garlic. Sauté for 3 to 5 minutes, or until the vegetables have started to soften.

4. Add the salt, pepper, red pepper flakes, and tomato paste. Cook, stirring, for 1 to 2 minutes to combine.

5. Add the tomato and then the wine. Cook, stirring occasionally, for 2 to 3 minutes, or until the wine has reduced by half.

6. Add the stock, and bring to a simmer. Cook for 5 to 7 minutes, or until the carrot is tender.

7. Add the clams, mussels, and salmon.

8. Reduce the heat to low. Cover the pot, and cook at a low simmer for 7 to 9 minutes, or until the clams and mussels have opened and the salmon is opaque and cooked through. Remove from the heat.

9. Garnish with the parsley and lemon.

Per Serving: Calories: 229; Total fat: 9g; Saturated fat: 1g; Protein: 16g; Total carbohydrates: 13g; Fiber: 3g; Sugar: 6g; Cholesterol: 38g

→ **VARIATION:** You can serve this dish with different types of fish, swapping out the salmon for halibut or rockfish. You can add 4 ounces raw scallops or shrimp with the other seafood ingredients in step 7 for added variety, flavor, and further antiangiogenic benefits.

Lemon-Thyme Salmon Meatballs

Dairy-Free, Gluten-Free,
Nut-Free, Soy-Free

SERVES 4

PREP TIME: 15 MINUTES / COOK TIME: 25 MINUTES

Classic meatballs get a new twist when they're made out of salmon. Plus,
they're much lower in saturated fat and higher in antiangiogenic omega-3's.
Serve these over whole-wheat pasta or greens for a balanced meal, or take
them to a party as an appetizer to share.

1 pound salmon, skin
   removed, cut into
   pieces, or 3 (5-ounce)
   cans salmon

1 tablespoon extra-virgin
   olive oil

½ medium yellow
   onion, diced

1 garlic clove, minced

¼ cup rolled oats

Zest and juice of 1 lemon

2 tablespoons chopped
   fresh thyme leaves

½ teaspoon dried
   oregano

¼ teaspoon dried dill

½ teaspoon salt

½ teaspoon freshly ground
   black pepper

1 egg

¼ cup chopped scallions,
   green and white parts

1. Preheat the oven to 350°F. Line a large sheet
   pan with parchment paper.

2. Put the salmon in a food processor, and
   pulse until finely chopped. (If you're using
   canned salmon, skip this step, and simply
   open and drain the cans instead. If you're
   using canned, cut the salt in half.) Transfer to
   a large mixing bowl.

3. In a large skillet, heat the oil over
   medium heat.

4. Add the onion and garlic. Sauté for 3 to
   5 minutes, or until soft and translucent.
   Remove from the heat. Transfer to the bowl
   with the salmon.

5. Add the oats, lemon zest and juice,
   thyme, oregano, dill, salt, pepper, and egg.
   Stir to combine.

6. Scoop out 2 tablespoons of the salmon
   mixture at a time, and using your hands, roll
   into a ball.

7. Place the meatballs, 1 inch apart, on the
   prepared sheet pan.

8. Transfer the sheet pan to the oven, and bake for 17 to 20 minutes, or until the meatballs are cooked through. They should be firm to the touch and golden brown. Remove from the oven.

9. Garnish with the scallions.

Per Serving: Calories: 252; Total fat: 12g; Saturated fat: 2g; Protein: 26g; Total carbohydrates: 9g; Fiber: 2g; Sugar: 1g; Cholesterol: 109g

→ **VARIATION:** You could also make these with tuna or whitefish. Add more spices or seasonings as desired; consider 1 tablespoon parsley or cilantro or ¼ teaspoon cayenne pepper.

Bioactive ingredients: salmon, olive oil, onion, garlic, oats, lemon, thyme, oregano

Anchovy Sourdough Toast with Capers

Dairy-Free, Nut-Free,
Soy-Free

SERVES 4

PREP TIME: 5 MINUTES / COOK TIME: 10 MINUTES

Anchovies are small, fatty fish that you eat with the bones, which makes them high in calcium. Don't worry at all; the bones are very soft in this type of fish. Serve anchovies on pieces of crusty sourdough toast—whether you make your own (see page 140) or purchase your favorite variety. Topped with salty, fermented capers, this dish is bursting with flavor and microbiome support.

4 (¼-inch-thick) sourdough bread slices

3 tablespoons extra-virgin olive oil, divided

2 tablespoons balsamic vinegar

¼ cup chopped fresh parsley

2 (2-ounce) cans anchovies

1 tablespoon capers

¼ cup olives, pitted and chopped

⅛ teaspoon red pepper flakes

Bioactive ingredients:
sourdough bread, olive oil, parsley, anchovy, capers

1. Preheat the oven to 350°F.

2. Put the bread on a sheet pan.

3. Drizzle with 1 tablespoon of oil.

4. Transfer the sheet pan to the oven, and bake for 10 minutes, or until toasted. Remove from the oven.

5. Meanwhile, to make the dressing, in a small mixing bowl, whisk together the vinegar, parsley, and remaining 2 tablespoons of oil.

6. Top the toasted bread with the anchovies, capers, olives, and red pepper flakes.

7. Drizzle with the dressing.

Per Serving: Calories: 299; Total fat: 13g; Saturated fat: 2g; Protein: 9g; Total carbohydrates: 35g; Fiber: 2g; Sugar: 4g; Cholesterol: 7g

→ **VARIATION:** You can try other fish in this recipe, like smoked salmon or sardines. Use whatever type of olives you enjoy the most: consider green, black, or Kalamata for slight variations on textures and flavors.

Miso-Honey Baked Mackerel

Dairy-Free, Nut-Free

SERVES 4

PREP TIME: 5 MINUTES / COOK TIME: 10 MINUTES

A versatile fish with a rich flavor, mackerel is an often-underutilized sustainable seafood option and a source of omega-3 fatty acids. This recipe takes the anti-angiogenic properties of fatty fish and adds a flavorful miso glaze for savory flavor and microbiome support. You can serve this dish over greens or with a side of your favorite whole grain, such as quinoa, farro, or barley, and vegetables for a complete meal.

2 tablespoons miso

1 tablespoon honey

1 tablespoon low-sodium soy sauce

1 tablespoon rice vinegar

1 tablespoon water

1 large shallot, finely chopped

4 (8-ounce) fresh mackerel fillets

½ lemon, cut into wedges

1 cup watercress

Bioactive ingredients: miso, soy sauce, mackerel, lemon, watercress

1. Preheat the oven to 350°F. Line a sheet pan with parchment paper.

2. To make the glaze, in a small mixing bowl, whisk together the miso, honey, soy sauce, vinegar, water, and shallot.

3. Place the mackerel, skin-side down, on the prepared sheet pan.

4. Drizzle or brush a thin coat of the glaze on top of each fillet, pouring any extra over the mackerel so it's completely coated.

5. Transfer the sheet pan to the oven, and bake for 10 minutes, or until golden brown. Remove from the oven.

6. Garnish with the lemon wedges and watercress.

Per Serving: Calories: 278; Total fat: 5g; Saturated fat: 1g; Protein: 48g; Total carbohydrates: 8g; Fiber: 1g; Sugar: 5g; Cholesterol: 120g

→ **VARIATION:** If you can't find mackerel or want a substitution, consider bluefish, herring, trout, or tuna.

Herb and Tomato Barley with Sardines

Dairy-Free, Nut-Free,
Soy-Free

SERVES 4

PREP TIME: 10 MINUTES / COOK TIME: 50 MINUTES

Whole-grain, fiber-rich barley pairs perfectly with savory tomatoes and protein-packed sardines, which are low in mercury and high in omega-3 fatty acids. Make sure to use pot barley because it's unprocessed, unlike pearled barley, which has had some of the fiber and nutrients removed.

1 cup pot barley, rinsed

2½ cups water

2 tablespoons extra-virgin olive oil, divided

3 garlic cloves, minced

½ yellow onion, finely chopped

½ teaspoon paprika

1 teaspoon salt, divided

1 teaspoon freshly ground black pepper

Juice of 1 lemon

1 large tomato, chopped

1 tablespoon chopped fresh tarragon leaves

¼ cup chopped fresh parsley

1 (4-ounce) can sardines, drained and chopped

Bioactive ingredients:
barley, olive oil, garlic, onion, lemon, tomato, parsley, sardine

1. In a large saucepan, combine the barley and water. Bring to a boil over medium-high heat.

2. Reduce the heat to low. Cover the sauce-pan, and simmer for 45 minutes, or until the barley is tender yet still chewy and all (or most of) the water has been absorbed. Remove from the heat. Transfer to a large mixing bowl.

3. Meanwhile, in a large stockpot, heat 1 tablespoon of oil over medium heat.

4. Add the garlic, onion, paprika, salt, and pepper. Sauté for 8 to 10 minutes, or until tender and translucent. Remove from the heat. Stir into the bowl of barley.

5. Drizzle the lemon juice and remaining 1 tablespoon of oil over everything.

6. Gently stir in the tomato, tarragon, parsley, and sardines.

Per Serving: Calories: 318; Total fat: 11g; Saturated fat: 2g; Protein: 13g; Total carbohydrates: 44g; Fiber: 9g; Sugar: 3g; Cholesterol: 40g

→ **VARIATION:** Feel free to use farro instead of barley for an alternative grain. You can replace the sardines with canned tuna or chopped anchovies.

Trout with Yogurt-Dill Sauce

Gluten-Free, Nut-Free,
Soy-Free

SERVES 4

PREP TIME: 5 MINUTES / COOK TIME: 15 MINUTES

A simple, mild baked trout requires very few ingredients and can be prepared in minutes. Adding a bright sauce to the fish makes a weeknight dinner a little fancier. Serve the trout with rice or roasted potatoes and Garlic Bok Choy (page 113).

4 (4-ounce) trout fillets, rinsed and patted dry

2 tablespoons olive oil

1 tablespoon freshly squeezed lemon juice

1 teaspoon salt, divided

6 ounces nonfat plain Greek yogurt or nondairy yogurt

½ small cucumber, seeded and diced

1 small garlic clove, minced

1 teaspoon extra-virgin olive oil

½ teaspoon red wine vinegar

1 tablespoon chopped fresh dill

Bioactive ingredients: trout, olive oil, lemon, yogurt, garlic

1. Preheat the oven to 400°F.

2. Arrange the trout fillets in a single layer on a sheet pan.

3. Drizzle with the olive oil, followed by the lemon juice and ⅞ teaspoon of salt.

4. Transfer the sheet pan to the oven, and bake for 10 to 12 minutes, or until the fillets have cooked through and flake easily when tested with a fork. Remove from the oven.

5. Meanwhile, to make the sauce, in a medium mixing bowl, whisk together the yogurt, cucumber, garlic, extra-virgin olive oil, vinegar, dill, and remaining ⅛ teaspoon of salt.

6. Serve each fillet topped with a dollop of the sauce.

Per Serving: Calories: 235; Total fat: 13g; Saturated fat: 3g; Protein: 25g; Total carbohydrates: 3g; Fiber: 0g; Sugar: 2g; Cholesterol: 72g

→ **VARIATION:** If you don't have access to trout, consider using cod, bluefish, or farmed sunshine bass or striped bass instead. If you'd prefer a smoother texture to the dill sauce, you can blend it or pulse it in a food processor so it's smooth but still has the nutrients and flavor of cucumber.

Spicy Salmon "Burger" Patties

Nut-Free, Soy-Free

SERVES 4

PREP TIME: 10 MINUTES / COOK TIME: 20 MINUTES

Skip the beef, and try salmon burgers for a healthier fat balance and a unique flavor. They're perfect for busy weeknights when you're crunched for time or for an outdoor event where you need a healthy, yet easy, option. Serve these in lettuce wraps or on whole-grain buns with a side of potatoes and greens.

1 pound salmon, skin removed, cut into pieces

1 tablespoon Dijon mustard

1 tablespoon nonfat plain yogurt or nondairy yogurt

⅓ cup whole-wheat bread crumbs

½ shallot, coarsely chopped

2 garlic cloves, minced

Zest and juice of ½ lemon

¾ teaspoon cayenne pepper

1 teaspoon salt

½ teaspoon freshly ground black pepper

4 whole-wheat hamburger buns, toasted

4 pieces red-leaf lettuce

½ large tomato, sliced

½ red onion, thinly sliced

1 ripe avocado, pitted, peeled, and sliced

Bioactive ingredients: salmon, yogurt, whole-wheat bread crumbs and buns, garlic, lemon, red-leaf lettuce, tomato, onion, avocado

1. Preheat the oven to 450°F. Line a sheet pan with wax paper.

2. Put the salmon in a food processor, and pulse until finely chopped.

3. Add the mustard, yogurt, bread crumbs, shallot, garlic, lemon zest and juice, cayenne, salt, and pepper. Pulse until combined.

4. Divide the salmon mixture into 4 equal parts on the prepared sheet pan.

5. Using your hands, form each portion into a ball, then flatten gently into a patty.

6. Transfer the sheet pan to the oven, and bake for 10 minutes. Flip the patties, and bake for 5 to 10 minutes, or until the outsides are slightly browned and each patty reaches an internal temperature of 145°F. Remove from the oven.

7. Serve the salmon burgers on the buns with the lettuce, tomato, onion, and avocado.

Per Serving: Calories: 395; Total fat: 17g; Saturated fat: 3g; Protein: 29g; Total carbohydrates: 33g; Fiber: 8g; Sugar: 7g; Cholesterol: 63g

Sheet Pan Salmon with Curried Romanesco

Dairy-Free, Gluten-Free,
Nut-Free, Soy-Free

SERVES 4

PREP TIME: 15 MINUTES / COOK TIME: 40 MINUTES

Pop this entire meal onto a sheet pan, and bake it for a hands-off, time-saving dinner. The combination of omega-3-rich salmon, colorful potatoes, and romanesco creates a balanced, health-promoting meal. A little milder than traditional cauliflower, romanesco can be a nice substitution to mix up your vegetable intake.

1 head romanesco, cut into bite-size florets

3 medium purple potatoes, chopped

2½ tablespoons extra-virgin olive oil, divided

2 teaspoons curry powder

½ teaspoon ground cumin

¾ teaspoon salt, divided

¾ teaspoon freshly ground black pepper, divided

4 (4-ounce) skin-on salmon fillets

¼ teaspoon chili powder

Bioactive ingredients:
romanesco, purple potato, olive oil, cumin, salmon

1. Preheat the oven to 400°F. Line a sheet pan with aluminum foil.

2. In a large mixing bowl, combine the romanesco, potatoes, 1½ tablespoons of oil, curry powder, cumin, ½ teaspoon of salt, and ½ teaspoon of pepper. Using a wooden spoon, toss to coat.

3. Place the salmon fillets, skin-side down, in the middle of the prepared sheet pan.

4. Drizzle with the remaining 1 tablespoon of oil, ¼ teaspoon of salt, and ¼ teaspoon of pepper and the chili powder.

5. Spread the potatoes and romanesco out evenly around the fillets.

6. Transfer the sheet pan to the oven, and bake for 25 to 30 minutes, or until the fillets have cooked through and the vegetables are tender enough to be pierced easily with a fork. Remove from the oven.

Per Serving: Calories: 458; Total fat: 21g; Saturated fat: 5g; Protein: 30g; Total carbohydrates: 39g; Fiber: 8g; Sugar: 5g; Cholesterol: 57g

Arctic Char with Tomato Curry

Dairy-Free, Gluten-Free,
Nut-Free, Soy-Free

SERVES 4

PREP TIME: 10 MINUTES / COOK TIME: 30 MINUTES

Arctic char is a sustainable seafood option, but this recipe works well with a variety of firm fish options, so you can use what is available to you locally.

3 tablespoons coconut oil

1 (2-inch) piece fresh
    ginger, grated

2 garlic cloves, minced

1 teaspoon ground coriander

1 teaspoon turmeric

1 teaspoon ground cumin

3 cups cherry tomatoes

¼ cup coconut cream
    (from the top of a can of
    coconut milk)

½ teaspoon salt

4 (5-ounce) skinless Arctic
    char fillets, rinsed and
    patted dry

1 cup fresh basil leaves,
    torn, divided

Bioactive ingredients: ginger, garlic, turmeric, cumin, tomato, Arctic char, basil

1. In a medium skillet, heat the oil over medium heat.

2. Add the ginger and garlic. Cook, stirring often, for about 3 minutes, or until the garlic has started to soften.

3. Stir in the coriander, turmeric, and cumin. Cook for about 30 seconds, or until fragrant.

4. Add the tomatoes, and cook, stirring occasionally, for 12 to 15 minutes, or until most of the tomatoes burst open.

5. Stir in the coconut cream and salt until well combined.

6. Reduce the heat to medium-low. Nestle the Arctic char fillets into the skillet, pressing them gently into the sauce.

7. Sprinkle ½ cup of basil on the fish and sauce. Cover the skillet, and cook at a low simmer for 5 to 7 minutes, or until the fillets are cooked throughout and beginning to flake. Remove from the heat.

8. Serve the fillets in serving bowls with the curry sauce poured over the top.

9. Garnish with the remaining ½ cup of basil.

Per Serving: Calories: 335; Total fat: 21g; Saturated fat: 14g; Protein: 31g; Total carbohydrates: 7g; Fiber: 2g; Sugar: 3g; Cholesterol: 84g

Mushroom-Ginger Steamed Halibut

Dairy-Free, Nut-Free

SERVES 4

PREP TIME: 15 MINUTES / COOK TIME: 15 MINUTES

Light, flaky halibut is the perfect fish to steam with savory vegetables, herbs, and spices. This simple dish features a savory stock as the base, topped with fresh cabbage and mushrooms (try it with shiitake or oyster mushrooms). Serve it over a bed of whole-grain brown or wild rice or quinoa.

1 pound fresh halibut

1 teaspoon salt, divided

2 tablespoons white wine

2 tablespoons low-sodium soy sauce

1 tablespoon rice vinegar

½ teaspoon honey

1 teaspoon grated fresh ginger

1 cup water

⅓ medium head napa cabbage, chopped

1 cup mushrooms, chopped

1 tablespoon toasted sesame oil

2 scallions, green and white parts, thinly sliced

½ lemon, sliced

Bioactive ingredients:
halibut, white wine, soy sauce, ginger, cabbage, mushroom, onion, lemon

1. Cut the halibut into 4 equal pieces. Season with ½ teaspoon of salt.

2. In a large skillet, combine the wine, soy sauce, vinegar, honey, ginger, and water. Bring to a boil over medium-high heat.

3. Reduce the heat to low. Add the cabbage and mushrooms. Season with the remaining ½ teaspoon of salt.

4. Place the halibut on top of the vegetables. Cover the skillet, and steam for 8 to 10 minutes, or until the halibut is opaque, cooked through, and reaches an internal temperature of 145°F. Remove from the heat.

5. Drizzle the oil over the halibut.

6. Garnish with the scallions and lemon.

Per Serving: Calories: 167; Total fat: 5g; Saturated fat: 1g; Protein: 23g; Total carbohydrates: 7g; Fiber: 2g; Sugar: 4g; Cholesterol: 56g

→ **VARIATION:** Consider substituting another firm fish, such as salmon, bluefish, trout, or hake, for the halibut. If you prefer more spice, add a teaspoon of chili oil or chile pepper to the stock.

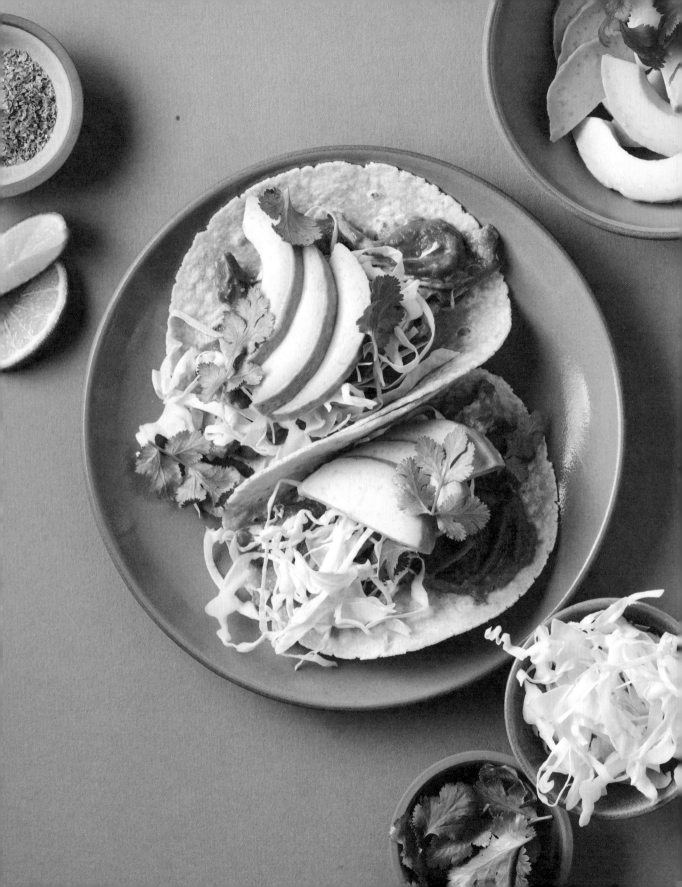

CHAPTER 6

Chicken

Chicken is so versatile and offers health benefits, especially from the dark meat, which has slightly more nutrients than white meat. I've included many variations on these recipes so you can mix and match to your preferences. You can even make many of these recipes vegetarian or vegan by swapping out the chicken for tofu or tempeh while still taking advantage of the many vibrant herbs, spices, fruits, vegetables, and whole grains that support your health throughout this chapter. You can also make many of them gluten-free by substituting tamari for soy sauce or gluten- and soy-free by substituting coconut aminos for soy sauce.

Chicken, Squash, and Kale Bowls with Pomegranate

Dairy-Free, Gluten-Free, Nut-Free, Soy-Free

SERVES 4

PREP TIME: 15 MINUTES / COOK TIME: 20 MINUTES, PLUS 10 MINUTES TO REST

A simple bowl balanced with protein-rich chicken, vibrant squash, and savory kale packs many health-promoting nutrients into one dish. The pomegranate garnish adds even more beautiful color, flavor, texture, and powerful anti-oxidant health benefits.

1 medium acorn squash, halved, seeded, and cut into ⅛-inch-thick pieces

5 tablespoons plus 1 teaspoon extra-virgin olive oil, divided

1 teaspoon salt, divided

¾ teaspoon freshly ground black pepper, divided

¼ teaspoon ground coriander

½ teaspoon ground cumin

¼ teaspoon ground cinnamon

4 boneless, skinless chicken thighs, trimmed

2 tablespoons freshly squeezed lemon juice

2 tablespoons white wine vinegar

2 teaspoons Dijon mustard

2 teaspoons maple syrup

2 tablespoons minced shallot

1 garlic clove, minced

1 teaspoon dried oregano

1 (5-ounce) package baby kale

1 cup pomegranate seeds

Bioactive ingredients: olive oil, cumin, cinnamon, chicken, lemon, garlic, oregano, kale, pomegranate

1. Preheat the oven to 450°F.

2. Spread the squash out on a sheet pan.

3. Drizzle 1 tablespoon of oil on top. Season the squash with ¼ teaspoon of salt and ¼ teaspoon of pepper.

4. Transfer the sheet pan to the oven, and roast for 10 to 13 minutes. Flip the squash, and roast for about 5 minutes, or until starting to brown and turn tender. Remove from the oven.

5. Meanwhile, in a small mixing bowl, whisk together 1 tablespoon of oil, ¼ teaspoon of salt, ¼ teaspoon of pepper, and the coriander, cumin, and cinnamon.

6. Put the chicken on another sheet pan.

7. Pour the olive oil and spice mixture on top, gently rubbing it onto the chicken.

8. Transfer the sheet pan to the oven, and bake for about 15 minutes, or until the chicken has cooked through and reaches an internal temperature of 165°F. Remove from the oven. Transfer the chicken to a cutting board. Let rest for 10 minutes, then slice.

9. While the squash and chicken are baking, to make the dressing, in a small bowl, combine the lemon juice, vinegar, mustard, maple syrup, shallot, garlic, oregano, and remaining 3 tablespoons and 1 teaspoon of oil, ½ teaspoon of salt, and ¼ teaspoon of pepper.

10. Divide the kale among 4 bowls.

11. Top with the squash, chicken, and pomegranate seeds.

12. Drizzle the dressing on top of each serving.

Per Serving: Calories: 411; Total fat: 27g; Saturated fat: 4g; Protein: 26g; Total carbohydrates: 27g; Fiber: 5g; Sugar: 9g; Cholesterol: 107g

→ **VARIATION:** For a vegetarian or vegan option, use tempeh instead of chicken, season it the same way, and roast it for the same amount of time. You can substitute the same amount of lettuce, arugula, or spinach for the kale to obtain similar health benefits but a different texture and flavor.

Chicken over Couscous with Honey-Lime-Tahini Dressing

Dairy-Free, Nut-Free	**SERVES 4**
	PREP TIME: 10 MINUTES / COOK TIME: 30 MINUTES, PLUS 10 MINUTES TO COOL

This easy dinner offers bright, zesty flavors combined with rich tahini dressing as a source of healthy fat that keeps you full and satisfied for hours. If you have one, use a cast-iron skillet or a Dutch oven. The benefit of a thick-bottomed pan or skillet is that you can both cook with it on the stove and also put it in the oven for finishing.

4 chicken thighs, trimmed and patted dry (about 1 pound)

2 garlic cloves, minced, divided

½ teaspoon paprika

¾ teaspoon salt

¼ teaspoon freshly ground black pepper

3 tablespoons extra-virgin olive oil, divided

1 cup whole-wheat pearl couscous

2 cups chicken stock or vegetable stock

2 tablespoons freshly squeezed lime juice

2 tablespoons tahini

1 tablespoon low-sodium soy sauce

1 teaspoon honey

¼ teaspoon red pepper flakes

2 tablespoons water

¼ cup fresh cilantro leaves

Bioactive ingredients: chicken, garlic, olive oil, whole-wheat couscous, tahini, soy sauce

1. Preheat the oven to 400°F.

2. Put the chicken on a large plate or platter.

3. In a small mixing bowl, combine half of the garlic, the paprika, the salt, the pepper, and 1 tablespoon of oil.

4. Sprinkle half of the mixture over the chicken, then flip and sprinkle with the remaining mixture.

5. In a large cast-iron skillet or oven-safe pot, heat 1 tablespoon of oil over medium-high heat.

6. Add the chicken, and cook for 3 to 5 minutes, or until golden brown. Transfer to a clean plate or platter.

7. In the same skillet, combine the remaining 1 tablespoon of oil, the remaining half of the garlic, and the couscous. Cook over medium-high heat, stirring frequently, for 2 to 3 minutes, or until the couscous is toasted.

8. Pour in the stock, and bring to a boil.

9. Return the chicken to the skillet. Turn off the heat.

10. Transfer the skillet to the oven, and bake for 15 minutes, or until the chicken has cooked through and the internal temperature has reached 165°F. Remove from the oven. Let cool for 5 to 10 minutes.

11. Meanwhile, to make the dressing, in a small mixing bowl, whisk together the lime juice, tahini, soy sauce, honey, red pepper flakes, and water.

12. Drizzle the dressing over the chicken and couscous.

13. Top with the cilantro.

Per Serving: Calories: 560; Total fat: 33g; Saturated fat: 7g; Protein: 26g; Total carbohydrates: 38g; Fiber: 3g; Sugar: 2g; Cholesterol: 111g

→ **VARIATION:** For alternative whole-grain options, you can prepare pearled millet, sorghum, quinoa, or brown rice, all of which are gluten-free options.

Fettuccine with Cilantro-Lime Chicken

Dairy-Free, Nut-Free

SERVES 4

PREP TIME: 15 MINUTES / COOK TIME: 25 MINUTES

This twist on chicken fettuccine alfredo lightens up the classic and is naturally dairy-free, relying on some coconut cream for the consistency. This dish is full of fresh vegetables and heat from a jalapeño, and the lime juice and cilantro add unexpected flavor and many health benefits, too.

12 ounces fettuccine

1½ pounds boneless, skinless chicken thighs, trimmed and diced

¾ teaspoon salt, divided

¾ teaspoon freshly ground black pepper, divided

2 tablespoons extra-virgin olive oil

1 cup sliced mushrooms

2 bell peppers, seeded and sliced

1 medium red onion, sliced

3 garlic cloves, minced

1 small jalapeño, seeded and diced

2 cups chicken stock

Juice of 1 lime

2 tablespoons low-sodium soy sauce

¼ cup coconut cream (from the top of a can of coconut milk)

1 teaspoon cornstarch

½ cup chopped fresh cilantro

1 lime, cut into wedges

Bioactive ingredients: chicken, olive oil, mushroom, bell pepper, onion, garlic, chile, soy sauce

1. Fill a large stockpot two-thirds full of water. Bring to a boil over high heat.

2. Add the fettuccine, and cook according to the package instructions (usually 10 to 12 minutes). Remove from the heat. Drain.

3. Meanwhile, season the chicken with ½ teaspoon of salt and ½ teaspoon of pepper.

4. In a large skillet, heat the oil over medium heat.

5. Add the chicken, and sauté for 2 to 3 minutes, or until the outside has started to cook.

6. Add the mushrooms, bell peppers, and onion. Cook, stirring frequently, for 5 to 7 minutes, or until the chicken has mostly cooked through and the vegetables have softened.

7. Add the garlic, jalapeño, and remaining ¼ teaspoon of salt and ¼ teaspoon of pepper. Cook, stirring frequently, for 1 minute.

8. Add the stock, lime juice, and soy sauce.

9. Increase the heat to medium-high. Simmer for 6 to 8 minutes, or until the flavors mingle.

10. Stir in the coconut cream. Return the sauce to a simmer, stirring occasionally to make sure the cream gets incorporated.

11. Transfer ¼ cup of the sauce to a small mixing bowl. Whisk the cornstarch into the bowl.

12. Return the mixture to the skillet, and stir. Cook for 2 to 3 minutes.

13. Add the fettuccine, and stir to coat. Remove from the heat.

14. Serve the pasta with the cilantro and lime wedges.

Per Serving: Calories: 685; Total fat: 21g; Saturated fat: 8g; Protein: 48g; Total carbohydrates: 77g; Fiber: 5g; Sugar: 4g; Cholesterol: 160g

→ **VARIATION:** If you don't like spice, you can eliminate the jalapeño. Instead, use any color of bell pepper that you enjoy, since they all contain health benefits, including the antioxidant vitamin C. You can also replace the cilantro with parsley if desired.

Hearty Braised Chicken Thighs with Sauerkraut

Dairy-Free, Gluten-Free, Nut-Free, Soy-Free

SERVES 4

PREP TIME: 10 MINUTES / COOK TIME: 40 MINUTES

This dish boosts gut health because of all the healthy fiber and natural probiotics. Refrigerated sauerkraut varieties will have more live probiotics than the shelf-stable variety, so head to the cold section to purchase your sauerkraut. Serve this dish with Brussels sprouts or a green salad and a whole grain like rice, quinoa, or barley.

3 tablespoons extra-virgin olive oil, divided

4 boneless, skinless chicken thighs, trimmed

1 teaspoon salt

1 teaspoon freshly ground black pepper

½ yellow onion, diced

1 medium carrot, diced

2 celery stalks, diced

1 medium Granny Smith apple, peeled, cored, and diced

2 cups sauerkraut, rinsed and drained

½ cup chicken stock

1 teaspoon Dijon mustard

2 teaspoons chopped fresh rosemary leaves

Bioactive ingredients: olive oil, chicken, onion, carrot, celery, apple, sauerkraut, rosemary

1. In a large skillet, heat 2 tablespoons of oil over medium-high heat.

2. Season the chicken with the salt and pepper. Add the chicken to the skillet. Cook for 2 to 3 minutes per side, or until golden brown. Transfer to a clean plate.

3. Reduce the heat to medium. In the same skillet, heat the remaining 1 tablespoon of oil.

4. Add the onion, carrot, celery, and apple. Cover the skillet, and cook for 5 minutes, or until starting to soften.

5. Stir in the sauerkraut, stock, mustard, rosemary, and chicken. Bring to a simmer.

6. Reduce the heat to low. Cover the skillet, and cook for 25 minutes, or until the chicken has reached an internal temperature of 165°F and most of the liquid is gone. Remove from the heat.

Per Serving: Calories: 281; Total fat: 15g; Saturated fat: 3g; Protein: 24g; Total carbohydrates: 12g; Fiber: 4g; Sugar: 7g; Cholesterol: 107g

Black Bean and Chicken Energy Bowls

Dairy-Free, Gluten-Free, Nut-Free, Soy-Free

SERVES 4

PREP TIME: 15 MINUTES / COOK TIME: 20 MINUTES

An energy bowl, or "power bowl," can be made from a variety of ingredients but should contain high-fiber whole grains, antioxidant-packed vegetables, plenty of protein, and lots of flavor. In this recipe, black beans and quinoa add fiber and protein; chicken offers vitamins, minerals, and more protein; and a variety of spices and vegetables offer unique flavors and antioxidants.

1 cup quinoa, rinsed

2 cups water

1 pound boneless, skinless chicken thighs, trimmed and patted dry

1 garlic clove, minced

½ teaspoon ground cumin

½ teaspoon salt

1 tablespoon extra-virgin olive oil

1 (15-ounce) can black beans, drained and rinsed

4 cups arugula

1 medium tomato, diced

1 ripe avocado, pitted, peeled, and sliced

Bioactive ingredients: quinoa, chicken, garlic, cumin, olive oil, beans, arugula, tomato, avocado

1. In a medium saucepan, combine the quinoa and water. Bring to a boil over high heat.

2. Reduce the heat to medium-low. Cover the saucepan, and cook for 15 minutes, or until the water has been absorbed and the quinoa is fluffy. Remove from the heat.

3. Meanwhile, cut the chicken into thin strips. Transfer to a medium mixing bowl.

4. Add the garlic, cumin, and salt to the bowl. Toss to combine.

5. In a large skillet, heat the oil over medium-high heat.

6. Add the chicken, and cook, stirring occasionally, for 5 minutes, or until lightly browned and cooked through.

7. Add the beans, and toss with the chicken to warm through. Remove from the heat.

8. Divide the quinoa among 4 bowls.

9. Top with the arugula, chicken, and beans, followed by the tomato and avocado.

Per Serving: Calories: 512; Total fat: 19g; Saturated fat: 4g; Protein: 37g; Total carbohydrates: 51g; Fiber: 14g; Sugar: 3g; Cholesterol: 107g

Maple-Garlic Chicken with Purple Potatoes

Dairy-Free, Nut-Free	**SERVES 4**
	PREP TIME: 10 MINUTES / COOK TIME: 45 TO 55 MINUTES

Sweet and savory, this simple chicken dish combines maple syrup, garlic, soy sauce, and onion, which offer unique health benefits that support all five defense systems. Using pantry items you likely already have on hand, this is a perfect busy weeknight dish. Serve it with a green salad on the side.

4 medium bone-in, skin-on chicken thighs, trimmed and patted dry

¾ teaspoon salt, divided

¾ teaspoon freshly ground black pepper, divided

3 tablespoons extra-virgin olive oil, divided

1 medium yellow onion, minced

1½ pounds purple potatoes, chopped

3 garlic cloves, minced

¼ cup maple syrup

1 tablespoon red wine vinegar

1 tablespoon low-sodium soy sauce

1 cup chopped broccoli

1 tablespoon fresh rosemary leaves, chopped, or 1 teaspoon dried rosemary, crumbled

1. Preheat the oven to 400°F.

2. Season the chicken with ½ teaspoon of salt and ½ teaspoon of pepper.

3. In a medium skillet, heat 2 tablespoons of oil over medium-high heat.

4. Place the chicken, skin-side down, in the skillet. Sear for 2 to 3 minutes per side, or until starting to brown. Transfer to a clean plate.

5. Add the onion and potatoes to the skillet. Sauté over medium-high heat for 8 to 10 minutes, or until golden brown and starting to soften. Transfer to a plate or bowl.

6. To make the sauce, add the remaining 1 tablespoon of oil to the skillet.

7. Reduce the heat to medium. Add the garlic, and sauté for about 1 minute, or until fragrant.

8. Add the maple syrup, vinegar, and soy sauce. Bring to a rolling simmer.

9. Reduce the heat to medium-low. Gently simmer for 3 to 5 minutes, or until the sauce has slightly thickened. Remove from the heat. Season with the remaining ¼ teaspoon of salt and ¼ teaspoon of pepper.

10. Reserve ⅓ cup of the sauce. Pour the remaining sauce into a roasting pan.

11. Add the potato mixture, and top with the broccoli.

12. Place the chicken thighs, skin-side up, on top of the broccoli.

13. Drizzle the reserved sauce over the chicken and broccoli.

14. Transfer the roasting pan to the oven, and bake for 20 to 30 minutes, or until the internal temperature of the chicken has reached 165°F. Remove from the oven.

15. Garnish with the rosemary, and serve warm.

Per Serving: Calories: 434; Total fat: 15g; Saturated fat: 3g; Protein: 27g; Total carbohydrates: 48g; Fiber: 5g; Sugar: 15g; Cholesterol: 107g

→ **VARIATION:** Garnishes can add extra flavor, color, and health benefits. Consider using parsley, thyme, or oregano instead of or in addition to the rosemary.

Chicken in Mango-Cashew Curry

Dairy-Free, Gluten-Free,
Soy-Free

SERVES 4

PREP TIME: 15 MINUTES, PLUS 8 HOURS TO
SOAK / COOK TIME: 35 MINUTES

Cashews are the secret ingredient in this dish. When they're soaked, then blended into a sauce, they create a rich, creamy, and health-promoting addition to the recipe. In order to be pureed, they need to be soaked for 8 hours or overnight. If you soak them for a shorter period of time, your sauce will just have larger pieces of cashew and be less creamy. Consider serving this dish over a bed of brown rice.

½ cup cashews

2 tablespoons extra-virgin
olive oil

2 bell peppers, seeded
and chopped

1 zucchini, cut into
half moons

½ large yellow onion, diced

2 garlic cloves, minced

1 (1-inch) piece fresh
ginger, grated

2 teaspoons curry powder

1 teaspoon turmeric

1 teaspoon salt

½ teaspoon freshly ground
black pepper

1½ tablespoons apple
cider vinegar

1 (13½-ounce) can light
coconut milk

2 mangos, peeled and
diced, divided

1½ pounds boneless,
skinless chicken thighs,
trimmed and diced

Bioactive ingredients: cashew,
olive oil, bell pepper, onion,
garlic, ginger, turmeric,
mango, chicken

1. Put the cashews in a medium saucepan, and cover with water. Soak for 8 hours or overnight.

2. After the cashews have soaked, to make the sauce, in a large pan, heat the oil over medium-high heat.

3. Add the bell peppers, zucchini, and onion. Sauté for 6 to 8 minutes, or until starting to soften.

4. Add the garlic and ginger. Sauté for about 1 minute, or until fragrant.

5. Stir in the curry powder, turmeric, salt, and pepper. Cook for 1 minute.

6. Add the vinegar, coconut milk, cashews, and half of the mango. Bring to a boil.

7. Reduce the heat to low. Simmer, stirring occasionally, for about 8 minutes, or until the sauce starts to thicken and the mango is very soft. Remove from the heat.

8. Pour the sauce into a blender, or keep it in the pan and use an immersion blender. Puree until smooth and creamy, then return the sauce to the pan.

9. Increase the heat to medium-high. Add the chicken, and bring to a simmer. Cover the pan, and cook for 10 minutes, or until the chicken has cooked through and reached an internal temperature of 165°F. Remove from the heat.

10. Stir in the remaining half of the mango.

Per Serving: Calories: 584; Total fat: 30g; Saturated fat: 10g; Protein: 40g; Total carbohydrates: 40g; Fiber: 6g; Sugar: 26g; Cholesterol: 160g

→ **VARIATION:** You can use 2 tablespoons curry paste instead of curry powder if that's your preference or what you have on hand. If you want to add a spicy kick to this dish, add 1 teaspoon red pepper flakes, which provides a nice balance to the sweet mango. If fresh mangos are not available in your area, you can thaw some frozen mango and use it instead.

Ginger Chicken and Vegetable Stir-Fry

Dairy-Free, Nut-Free	**SERVES 4**
	PREP TIME: 15 MINUTES, PLUS 15 MINUTES TO MARINATE / COOK TIME: 20 MINUTES

Stir-fry is such a perfect dish for maximizing your vegetable intake and getting creative in the kitchen. There are four hearty vegetables in this recipe that help promote both flavor and health, but you're free to weave in other options that you enjoy. This is a dish you can make again and again in slightly different variations. Even if you didn't enjoy a particular vegetable previously, a stir-fry can be a way to try it again. Consider serving this dish over brown or wild rice.

1 pound boneless, skinless chicken thighs, trimmed and cut into 1-inch pieces

2 scallions, green and white parts, thinly sliced

2 tablespoons honey

1 tablespoon sesame oil

1 tablespoon white wine vinegar

2 tablespoons low-sodium soy sauce, divided

3 garlic cloves, minced, divided

1 (½-inch) piece fresh ginger, peeled and minced, divided

¾ teaspoon salt

½ teaspoon freshly ground black pepper

3 tablespoons extra-virgin olive oil, divided

½ large yellow onion, diced

1 carrot, cut into rounds

1 cup chopped broccoli

2 bell peppers, seeded and chopped

1 tablespoon cornstarch

⅓ cup water

Bioactive ingredients: chicken, soy sauce, garlic, ginger, olive oil, onion, carrot, broccoli, bell pepper

1. In a large mixing bowl, combine the chicken, scallions, honey, sesame oil, vinegar, 1 tablespoon of soy sauce, half of the garlic, half of the ginger, the salt, and the pepper. Stir to coat the chicken. Marinate for 15 minutes.

2. Meanwhile, in a large pan, heat 2 tablespoons of olive oil over medium heat.

3. Add the onion, carrot, and broccoli. Cook for 2 to 4 minutes, or until starting to soften.

4. Add the bell peppers and the remaining half of the garlic and ginger. Stir-fry for 4 to 5 minutes, or until the vegetables have a vibrant color and are fork tender. Transfer to a plate.

5. In a small mixing bowl, mix together the cornstarch and water.

6. In the same skillet, heat the remaining 1 tablespoon of olive oil over medium heat.

7. Add the chicken, and cook for 3 to 4 minutes, or until browned on the outside but not cooked entirely through.

8. Add the remaining 1 tablespoon of soy sauce, and return the stir-fried vegetables to the skillet.

9. Pour in the cornstarch mixture, stirring to combine.

10. Increase the heat to medium-high. Bring to a simmer. Cook for 2 to 4 minutes, or until the mixture has thickened and the chicken is cooked through. Remove from the heat.

Per Serving: Calories: 347; Total fat: 19g; Saturated fat: 3g; Protein: 25g; Total carbohydrates: 21g; Fiber: 3g; Sugar: 13g; Cholesterol: 107g

→ **VARIATION:** For a vegetarian-friendly version, use chopped extra-firm tofu or tempeh in place of the chicken. This will provide protein and additional antioxidants. You could swap in or add vegetables such as green beans, snap peas, zucchini, or cauliflower if desired.

Whole Roasted Chicken and Root Vegetable Sheet Pan Dinner

Dairy-Free, Gluten-Free,
Nut-Free, Soy-Free

SERVES 6

PREP TIME: 20 MINUTES / COOK TIME: 1 HOUR 30 MINUTES

If you've got a family or roommates, or you simply enjoy having leftovers to make healthy eating later in the week easier, this is a great recipe to add to your repertoire. Simply season a whole chicken with plenty of fresh, health-promoting herbs and vibrant fresh lemon, then roast it on a sheet pan with a variety of hearty root vegetables. Keep prep simple by not peeling the carrots or turnips.

1 whole chicken,
    giblets removed

1½ teaspoons salt, divided

1 lemon, zested and cut
    into wedges

1 celery stalk, chopped

3 large rosemary sprigs

3 sage sprigs

2 sweet potatoes, peeled
    and chopped

4 medium red beets, peeled
    and chopped

4 medium carrots, unpeeled,
    cut into rounds

2 medium turnips, unpeeled,
    cut into rounds

1 yellow onion, cut
    into wedges

2 tablespoons extra-virgin
    olive oil

5 garlic cloves, minced

½ teaspoon freshly ground
    black pepper

Bioactive ingredients: chicken, lemon, celery, rosemary, sage, sweet potato, beet, carrot, turnip, onion, olive oil, garlic

1. Preheat the oven to 350°F.

2. Season the chicken with 1 teaspoon of salt and the lemon zest, using your hands to rub them onto the skin.

3. Stuff the lemon wedges, celery, rosemary, and sage into the chicken cavity.

4. Spread the sweet potatoes, beets, carrots, turnips, and onion out on a large sheet pan, keeping the middle somewhat cleared for the chicken.

5. Drizzle with the oil, then sprinkle with the garlic, the remaining ½ teaspoon of salt, and the pepper. Stir to coat.

6. Place the chicken in the middle of the sheet pan.

7. Transfer the sheet pan to the oven, and roast for 1 hour 30 minutes, or until the vegetables are soft and the chicken has reached an internal temperature of 165°F. Remove from the oven.

Per Serving: Calories: 519; Total fat: 29g; Saturated fat: 7g; Protein: 41g; Total carbohydrates: 23g; Fiber: 5g; Sugar: 10g; Cholesterol: 168g

→ **VARIATION:** You can use different types of root vegetables if you desire. Swap out the sweet potatoes for 2 or 3 chopped red or purple potatoes. Use golden beets instead of red beets. Consider using parsnips or rutabagas instead of the carrots or turnips. You can also use a red onion instead of yellow.

Dark-Meat Chicken Stew with Barley

Dairy-Free, Nut-Free,
Soy-Free

SERVES 4

PREP TIME: 15 MINUTES / COOK TIME: 1 HOUR

You should have a rich stew in your arsenal, and this one helps you easily meet your daily vegetable and fiber intake. Dark-meat chicken provides protein and minerals like zinc and iron, while barley, an often-underutilized whole grain, boosts the fiber and B vitamins in this dish. Toss in some spinach and fresh lemon at the end for a bright, zesty addition to a very savory stew.

1 pound boneless, skinless chicken thighs, rinsed and patted dry

1½ teaspoons salt, divided

1 teaspoon freshly ground black pepper, divided

2 tablespoons extra-virgin olive oil, divided

1 yellow onion, diced

2 medium carrots, diced

2 celery stalks, diced

3 garlic cloves, minced

¼ cup water, divided

3 red potatoes, diced

6 cups chicken stock or vegetable stock

1 cup barley

1 teaspoon dried thyme

1 teaspoon dried rosemary

1 teaspoon dried sage

1 cup chopped spinach

Juice of 1 lemon

1. Season the chicken with ¾ teaspoon of salt and ¾ teaspoon of pepper, rubbing it in to coat evenly.

2. In a large stockpot or Dutch oven, heat 1 tablespoon of oil over medium heat.

3. Add the chicken, cover the pot, and cook for 5 to 6 minutes per side, or until the chicken is cooked through and the internal temperature has reached 165°F. Transfer to a large mixing bowl. Shred using 2 forks, or a fork and a knife, moving in opposite directions.

4. In the same pot, warm the remaining 1 tablespoon of oil over medium heat.

5. Add the onion, carrots, celery, ¼ teaspoon of salt, and the remaining ¼ teaspoon of pepper. Sauté for 5 to 6 minutes, or until starting to soften.

6. Add the garlic, and sauté for 30 seconds, or until fragrant.

7. Add the water, 1 tablespoon at a time, and stir to loosen any ingredients that are sticking to the pot.

8. Add the potatoes, stock, barley, thyme, rosemary, sage, and remaining ½ teaspoon of salt.

9. Increase the heat to medium-high. Bring the liquid to a boil.

10. Reduce the heat to medium-low. Cover the pot, and simmer for 20 minutes.

11. Return the chicken to the pot. Cook, covered, for 10 minutes, or until the potatoes are soft enough to pierce with a fork and the barley is tender.

12. Add the spinach, and cook for 1 to 2 minutes, or until just wilted.

13. Add the lemon juice. Remove from the heat.

Per Serving: Calories: 517; Total fat: 12g; Saturated fat: 2g; Protein: 31g; Total carbohydrates: 72g; Fiber: 13g; Sugar: 5g; Cholesterol: 107g

→ **VARIATION:** You can replace the barley with different grains, such as buckwheat groats, farro, or wild rice. Consider swapping in a rutabaga, turnip, or 2 parsnips for the carrots. You can use beet greens, mustard greens, collard greens, or Swiss chard instead of or in addition to the spinach.

Bioactive ingredients: chicken, olive oil, onion, carrot, celery, garlic, barley, thyme, rosemary, sage, spinach, lemon

Sheet Pan Citrus Chicken with Brussels Sprouts

Dairy-Free, Gluten-Free, Nut-Free, Soy-Free

SERVES 4

PREP TIME: 15 MINUTES, PLUS AT LEAST 1 HOUR TO MARINATE / COOK TIME: 40 MINUTES

This unexpected flavor combination brings savory roast chicken thighs together with garlic, bright lime juice, spicy jalapeño, and fresh mint. The marinade is versatile and can be used with other meats, on plant-based proteins like tofu or tempeh, or even as a salad dressing. Enjoy this dish on its own, or consider serving it over brown or wild rice or quinoa.

FOR THE MARINADE

Grated zest of ½ orange

Juice of 1 orange

Grated zest of 1 lime

Juice of 2 limes

2 garlic cloves

¼ cup extra-virgin olive oil

½ jalapeño, seeded

½ teaspoon salt

¼ teaspoon freshly ground black pepper

5 fresh mint leaves

FOR THE CHICKEN AND BRUSSELS SPROUTS

8 small bone-in, skin-on chicken thighs

¾ teaspoon salt, divided

½ teaspoon freshly ground black pepper, divided

4 cups (about 1 pound) Brussels sprouts, halved

2 tablespoons extra-virgin olive oil

1 garlic clove, minced

1 orange, cut into rounds

Bioactive ingredients: orange, garlic, olive oil, chile, mint, chicken

TO MAKE THE MARINADE

1. In a blender or food processor, combine the orange zest, orange juice, lime zest, lime juice, garlic, oil, jalapeño, salt, pepper, and mint. Puree until smooth.

2. Pour ¼ cup of the marinade into a large mixing bowl, and reserve the rest in the refrigerator in a covered bowl or jar.

TO MAKE THE CHICKEN AND BRUSSELS SPROUTS

3. Season the chicken with ½ teaspoon of salt and ¼ teaspoon of pepper.

4. Put the chicken in the large bowl with the marinade. Using your hands, rub the marinade over the chicken until completely coated. Cover, and refrigerate for 1 hour or up to 4 hours.

5. When you're ready to cook the chicken, remove from the refrigerator. Preheat the oven to 450°F.

6. Spread the Brussels sprouts out on a large sheet pan.

7. Drizzle with the oil, and sprinkle with the garlic, remaining ¼ teaspoon of salt, and remaining ¼ teaspoon of pepper.

8. Nestle the chicken pieces, skin-side up, among the Brussels sprouts.

9. Drizzle the reserved marinade over everything.

10. Arrange the orange slices on top of the chicken and Brussels sprouts.

11. Transfer the sheet pan to the oven, and roast for 35 to 40 minutes, or until the chicken is browned and crisp and has reached an internal temperature of 165°F. Remove from the oven.

Per Serving: Calories: 277; Total fat: 15g; Saturated fat: 3g; Protein: 26g; Total carbohydrates: 10g; Fiber: 4g; Sugar: 3g; Cholesterol: 107g

→ **VARIATION:** You can use other vegetables in addition to or instead of the Brussels sprouts. Consider delicata, butternut, or patty pan squash; potatoes; carrots; or parsnips.

Chicken Tinga Tacos

Dairy-Free, Gluten-Free,
Nut-Free, Soy-Free

SERVES 4 (12 TACOS)

PREP TIME: 15 MINUTES / COOK TIME: 20 MINUTES

This dish is inspired by chicken tinga, or *tinga de pollo* in Spanish, a Mexican dish of shredded chicken cooked in a tomato sauce with savory spices like oregano and cumin. In this version, the meat is served street taco–style on small corn tortillas and garnished with health-promoting, colorful vegetables for a balanced lunch or dinner. Add a simple green salad or a side of beans for even more fiber and protein.

1½ pounds boneless, skinless chicken thighs, trimmed

3½ cups chicken stock, divided

1 tablespoon extra-virgin olive oil

½ cup chopped yellow onion

2 garlic cloves, minced

1 teaspoon dried oregano

½ teaspoon ground cumin

½ teaspoon cayenne pepper

1 (15-ounce) can crushed fire-roasted tomatoes

½ teaspoon salt

12 (6-inch) corn tortillas

1 large ripe avocado, sliced

1 cup shredded cabbage

¼ cup chopped fresh cilantro

1. In a large stockpot, combine the chicken and 3 cups of stock. (The meat should be covered by about an inch of stock. Depending on the size of your pot, you may need to add water to cover the chicken properly.) Bring to a boil over medium-high heat.

2. Reduce the heat to medium. Simmer for 10 to 12 minutes, or until the chicken has cooked through and the internal temperature has reached 165°F. Remove from the heat. Using tongs, transfer to a large mixing bowl. Using 2 forks, pull the meat apart in opposite directions until completely shredded.

3. Meanwhile, in a large skillet, heat the oil over medium heat.

4. Add the onion, and cook for about 4 minutes, or until translucent.

5. Add the garlic, and cook for 30 seconds, or until fragrant.

6. Stir in the oregano, cumin, and cayenne. Cook for 30 seconds, or until fragrant.

7. Add the tomatoes, salt, and remaining ½ cup of stock.

8. Increase the heat to medium-high. Bring the sauce to a simmer. Cook for 3 to 4 minutes, or until slightly thickened. Remove from the heat.

9. Carefully pour the sauce into a blender, and blend until smooth. (You can also use an immersion blender to blend it in the skillet.)

10. Return the sauce to the skillet, and stir in the shredded chicken to coat. Cook over low heat for 2 to 3 minutes, or until the flavors meld. Remove from the heat.

11. Serve the chicken in the sauce on top of the tortillas.

12. Garnish each taco with the avocado, cabbage, and cilantro.

Per Serving: Calories: 530; Total fat: 20g; Saturated fat: 4g; Protein: 41g; Total carbohydrates: 51g; Fiber: 12g; Sugar: 7g; Cholesterol: 160g

Bioactive ingredients: chicken, onion, garlic, oregano, cumin, tomato, avocado, cabbage

→ **INGREDIENT TIP:** You can save time by using cooked chicken. Simply start at step 3. Just make sure that the chicken is fully heated through in step 10. Consider adding cheese as a garnish if desired; shredded Gouda adds antiangiogenic and microbiome support.

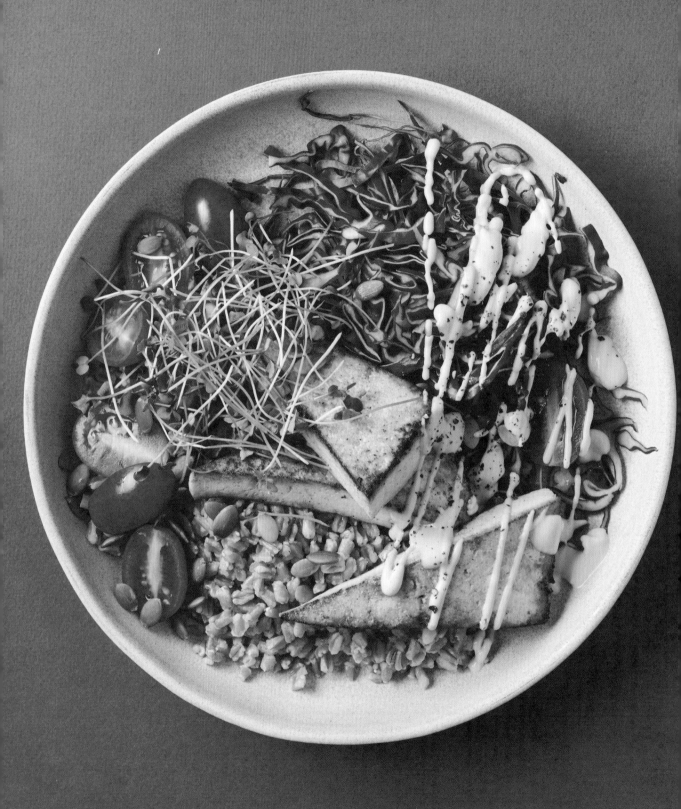

CHAPTER 7

Vegetarian Mains and Sides

Most of us know that we should be eating more vegetables. According to the Centers for Disease Control and Prevention, only 1 in 10 US adults consumes enough fresh produce. Making vegetables a regular part of your daily diet and knowing how to prepare them in a variety of delicious ways are both keys to success. The recipes in this chapter are simple and versatile; swap in other favorite vegetables, herbs, and spices as needed to make each one your own. Don't forget to experiment with new options as well; you may be surprised that vegetables you didn't previously care for are appealing when prepared in a different way. Many vegetables help support most, if not all, of the five defense systems, so they're a key food group to get familiar and comfortable with.

Endive and Chickpea Bites

Gluten-Free, Nut-Free,
Soy-Free, Vegetarian

SERVES 4

PREP TIME: 15 MINUTES

An often-underutilized vegetable, endive is actually a part of the chicory family, like radicchio, escarole, and frisée. These vegetables are known for their slightly bitter flavor, which provides a nice contrast to other vegetables, herbs, and spices. These appetizer-size bites are perfect for a party, snack, or simple lunch.

2 tablespoons nonfat plain Greek yogurt or nondairy yogurt

½ tablespoon maple syrup

Grated zest and juice of 1 small lemon

½ teaspoon salt

¼ teaspoon freshly ground black pepper

1 medium apple, cored and diced

½ (15-ounce) can chickpeas, drained and rinsed well

¼ cup finely chopped celery

¼ cup thinly sliced scallion, green and white parts

½ cup chopped fresh parsley

8 Belgian endive leaves (about 2 heads)

Bioactive ingredients: yogurt, lemon, apple, beans, celery, onion, parsley, Belgian endive

1. In a large bowl, mix together the yogurt, maple syrup, lemon zest, lemon juice, salt, and pepper.

2. Add the apple, chickpeas, celery, scallions, and parsley. Stir to coat evenly.

3. Spoon the mixture into each of the endive leaves.

4. Arrange the endive boats on a platter to serve.

Per Serving: Calories: 100; Total fat: 4g; Saturated fat: 0g; Protein: 1g; Total carbohydrates: 20g; Fiber: 7g; Sugar: 9g; Cholesterol: 1g

→ **VARIATION:** You can substitute vegan or regular mayonnaise for yogurt, and you can substitute navy beans for chickpeas for a softer texture. For a different flavor, swap in cilantro for the parsley, or use other health-promoting herbs like rosemary, oregano, or thyme.

Lemony White Bean Dip

Dairy-Free, Gluten-Free, Nut-Free, Soy-Free, Vegan

SERVES 4

PREP TIME: 5 MINUTES

A simple bean dip is a savory, protein-packed, and health-promoting snack that kids and adults can enjoy every day. This recipe is no-cook and can be made in minutes in a blender or food processor. It's great paired with a variety of fresh vegetables but can also be used as a spread on a sandwich or wrap.

1 (15-ounce) can cannellini, navy, or great northern beans, drained and rinsed

1½ tablespoons extra-virgin olive oil

Grated zest and juice of 1 small lemon

1 garlic clove

½ teaspoon salt

¼ teaspoon freshly ground black pepper

4 tablespoons water, divided

4 fresh basil leaves

2 parsley sprigs

Bioactive ingredients: beans, olive oil, lemon, garlic, basil, parsley

1. Put the beans, oil, lemon zest, lemon juice, garlic, salt, pepper, and 2 tablespoons of water in a food processor or blender. Pulse until completely combined.

2. Add the remaining 2 tablespoons of water, 1 tablespoon at a time, to achieve your desired creamy consistency.

3. Add the basil and parsley. Pulse 4 to 5 more times to incorporate the herbs without blending them in completely, so that pieces of the leaves are visible.

Per Serving: Calories: 127; Total fat: 5g; Saturated fat: 1g; Protein: 6g; Total carbohydrates: 15g; Fiber: 5g; Sugar: 0g; Cholesterol: 0g

→ **VARIATION:** All beans are beneficial due to their high fiber and protein content in addition to their vitamins, minerals, and unique antioxidants. You can make this dip with chickpeas for more of a hummus-style dip, or you could get creative with black or pinto beans.

Basil-Kimchi Fried Rice

Dairy-Free, Nut-Free, Vegan

SERVES 4

PREP TIME: 10 MINUTES / COOK TIME: 20 MINUTES

Fried rice gets a nutritional boost when you add savory, spicy kimchi to it. This fermented cabbage is a source of the good bacteria that have been shown to promote microbiome health.

2 tablespoons extra-virgin olive oil

½ yellow onion, diced

2 medium carrots, diced

2 garlic cloves, minced

½ cup chopped fresh basil leaves, divided

1 teaspoon dried thyme

¼ teaspoon salt

½ teaspoon freshly ground black pepper

1 cup frozen green peas, thawed

½ cup frozen edamame, thawed

2 cups cooked brown rice

¼ cup low-sodium soy sauce

¼ cup vegan kimchi

Bioactive ingredients:
olive oil, onion, carrot, garlic, basil, thyme, peas, edamame, brown rice, soy sauce, kimchi

1. In a large skillet, heat the oil over medium-high heat.

2. Add the onion, and sauté for 2 to 3 minutes, or until starting to soften.

3. Add the carrots, and continue to sauté for 5 to 7 minutes, or until tender.

4. Add the garlic, ¼ cup of basil, and the thyme, salt, and pepper. Heat for about 1 minute, or until fragrant.

5. Stir in the peas and edamame. Cook for 3 to 5 minutes, or until heated through.

6. Add the rice, and fold the vegetables into the rice until they are well distributed throughout. Cook for 1 to 3 minutes, or until the rice is heated through.

7. Add the soy sauce, and stir into the rice until incorporated. Remove from the heat.

8. Add the kimchi and remaining ¼ cup of basil.

Per Serving: Calories: 250; Total fat: 9g; Saturated fat: 1g; Protein: 8g; Total carbohydrates: 35g; Fiber: 6g; Sugar: 5g; Cholesterol: 0g

→ **VARIATION:** For more protein, add cooked tempeh, tofu, or dark-meat chicken at the end before serving. Add red chiles or red pepper flakes if you want more heat.

Garlic Bok Choy

Dairy-Free, Nut-Free, Vegan

SERVES 4

PREP TIME: 5 MINUTES / COOK TIME: 15 MINUTES

Bok choy is a delicious, delicate member of the cruciferous family. Pair this dish with baked tofu or tempeh and rice, or serve it as a side to one of the many fish or seafood recipes in this book.

1 tablespoon extra-virgin olive oil

3 garlic cloves, minced

2 pounds baby bok choy, halved (quartered if very large), keeping the leaves attached at the base

1 tablespoon low-sodium soy sauce

1 tablespoon water

1 teaspoon red pepper flakes

Bioactive ingredients: olive oil, garlic, bok choy, soy sauce

1. In a large skillet, heat the oil over medium-high heat.

2. Add the garlic, and cook, stirring continuously, for 1 to 2 minutes, or until fragrant and lightly browned.

3. Add the bok choy, and stir to coat the leaves as best you can.

4. Sprinkle the soy sauce and water evenly over the greens, then cover the skillet. Cook for 2 to 3 minutes.

5. Stir gently, then cover the skillet again. Cook for 8 to 10 minutes, or until the stalks have softened and the tops have wilted. Remove from the heat.

6. Sprinkle with the red pepper flakes.

Per Serving: Calories: 65; Total fat: 4g; Saturated fat: 1g; Protein: 4g; Total carbohydrates: 6g; Fiber: 2g; Sugar: 3g; Cholesterol: 0g

→ **VARIATION:** You can add more garlic, if desired; for even more health benefits and a stronger flavor, consider 1 clove more. Feel free to eliminate the red pepper flakes completely or replace with ½ teaspoon freshly ground black pepper for a less spicy dish.

Savory Roasted Cauliflower

Dairy-Free, Gluten-Free,
Nut-Free, Soy-Free, Vegan

SERVES 5

PREP TIME: 5 MINUTES / COOK TIME: 25 MINUTES

Whether it's white, purple, green, or any other color, cauliflower is anti-angiogenic, supports the microbiome, and helps protect DNA and the immune system. Get creative by choosing your favorite color of cauliflower or even replacing it with the slightly milder romanesco. Part of the cruciferous vegetable family, cauliflower contains sulfuric compounds that have shown to be beneficial to human health in a variety of ways (Manchali et al. 2012).

2 tablespoons extra-virgin olive oil

1 small head cauliflower, cut into florets

½ teaspoon salt

⅛ teaspoon freshly ground black pepper

1 garlic clove, minced

¼ teaspoon chili powder

½ teaspoon ground cumin

2 teaspoons fresh thyme leaves, chopped

Bioactive ingredients: olive oil, cauliflower, garlic, cumin, thyme

1. Preheat the oven to 450°F. Line a sheet pan with aluminum foil or a silicone liner.

2. In a large mixing bowl, combine the oil and cauliflower. Season with the salt, pepper, garlic, chili powder, and cumin.

3. Pour the mixture onto the prepared sheet pan, scraping any additional oil and spices out of the bowl and onto the cauliflower.

4. Transfer the sheet pan to the oven, and roast for 10 to 12 minutes. Flip the cauliflower, and roast for 10 to 13 minutes, or until tender. Remove from the oven.

5. Garnish with the thyme.

Per Serving: Calories: 79; Total fat: 7g; Saturated fat: 1g; Protein: 1g; Total carbohydrates: 4g; Fiber: 2g; Sugar: 1g; Cholesterol: 0g

→ **VARIATION:** Consider adding more garlic if desired; another 1 or 2 cloves will create a stronger flavor. You could also swap the thyme leaves out for 1 tablespoon parsley or cilantro.

Citrus-Herb Asparagus

Dairy-Free, Gluten-Free, Nut-Free, Soy-Free, Vegan

SERVES 4

PREP TIME: 5 MINUTES / COOK TIME: 20 MINUTES

A perfect side for any meal, this quick and easy asparagus recipe will become a staple in your home. It is crisp and vibrant with health-promoting properties from fresh citrus and herbs, like parsley. Having go-to recipes for vegetables that you really enjoy boosts the chances that they'll become a regular part of your diet.

2 tablespoons extra-virgin olive oil

1 tablespoon freshly squeezed lemon juice

1 garlic clove, minced

1 teaspoon dried oregano

1 teaspoon dried rosemary

1 teaspoon dried parsley

⅛ teaspoon salt

¼ teaspoon freshly ground black pepper

1 pound asparagus spears, woody ends trimmed

1 teaspoon chopped fresh chives or scallions

Bioactive ingredients: olive oil, lemon, garlic, oregano, rosemary, parsley, asparagus, onion

1. Preheat the oven to 350°F. Line a sheet pan with parchment paper.

2. In a small mixing bowl, whisk together the oil, lemon juice, garlic, oregano, rosemary, parsley, salt, and pepper.

3. Arrange the asparagus in a single layer on the prepared sheet pan.

4. Drizzle with the oil and herb mixture, then toss to coat.

5. Transfer the sheet pan to the oven, and roast for 10 to 20 minutes, or until the asparagus is tender and lightly browned. Remove from the oven.

6. Garnish with the chives.

Per Serving: Calories: 85; Total fat: 7g; Saturated fat: 1g; Protein: 3g; Total carbohydrates: 5g; Fiber: 3g; Sugar: 2g; Cholesterol: 0g

→ **VARIATION:** This preparation can also work well with squash, Brussels sprouts, or broccoli. You may need to extend the cooking time by 5 or 10 minutes for other vegetables.

Herb-Stuffed Mushrooms

Nut-Free, Soy-Free,
Vegetarian

SERVES 6

PREP TIME: 15 MINUTES / COOK TIME: 40 MINUTES

Stuffed mushrooms are a treat, but some similar recipes make a heavy dish that is high in saturated fat. I'm happy to report that you can easily lighten them up to benefit your health with natural, flavorful ingredients. Small, bite-size options like Baby Bellas or white mushrooms are easy to stuff with whole-wheat bread crumbs, savory Parmigiano-Reggiano cheese, and lots of fresh and dried herbs.

24 white mushrooms

2 tablespoons extra-virgin olive oil

½ yellow onion, diced

2 tablespoons dry white wine

½ cup whole-wheat panko bread crumbs

1 egg, beaten

2 teaspoons chopped fresh chives, divided

2 teaspoons chopped fresh parsley, divided

2 teaspoons dried oregano, divided

¾ teaspoon salt

½ teaspoon freshly ground black pepper

4 tablespoons freshly grated Parmigiano-Reggiano cheese, divided

1. Preheat the oven to 350°F. Line a sheet pan with parchment paper.

2. Remove and finely chop the mushroom stems. Place the mushroom caps, upside down, on the prepared sheet pan.

3. In a medium skillet, heat the oil over medium-high heat.

4. Add the chopped mushroom stems and the onion. Sauté for 2 to 4 minutes, or until starting to soften.

5. Add the wine, and cook for 2 minutes, or until the mushrooms are soft and incorporated. Remove from the heat. Transfer the vegetables to a medium mixing bowl.

6. Stir in the bread crumbs. Let cool for 5 minutes.

7. To make the filling, add the egg, 1½ teaspoons of chives, 1½ teaspoons of parsley, 1½ teaspoons of oregano, and the salt, pepper, and 2 tablespoons of cheese. Stir well to combine.

8. Spoon the filling into each of the mush-
    room caps, so that the filling is slightly
    rounded on the top.

9. Sprinkle the remaining 2 tablespoons of
    cheese on top.

10. Transfer the sheet pan to the oven, and bake
    for 30 minutes, or until the mushrooms are
    tender and the tops are browned. Remove
    from the oven. Let cool slightly.

11. Garnish with the remaining ½ teaspoon
    of chives, ½ teaspoon of parsley, and
    ½ teaspoon of oregano.

Per Serving: Calories: 120; Total fat: 7g; Saturated fat: 2g;
Protein: 5g; Total carbohydrates: 10g; Fiber: 1g; Sugar: 2g;
Cholesterol: 30g

→ **VARIATION:** You can mix up the herbs in these
    savory mushrooms by swapping in or adding
    1 teaspoon sage or basil. Add smoky and spicy
    flavors with ¼ teaspoon smoked paprika, cay-
    enne, or chili powder.

Bioactive ingredients:
mushroom, olive oil,
onion, white wine,
whole-wheat bread
crumbs, parsley, oregano,
Parmigiano-Reggiano

Green Cauliflower Rice with Baked Tofu

Dairy-Free, Gluten-Free, Nut-Free, Vegan	SERVES 4
	PREP TIME: 10 MINUTES / COOK TIME: 30 MINUTES

Cauliflower "rices" very well: you can either grate it or finely chop it in a food processor yourself. Or you can purchase it as frozen "rice." This version is complemented by fresh herbs and topped with baked tofu. The tofu can be prepared on its own and eaten as a simple snack or added to a salad or sandwich for extra protein.

1 teaspoon coconut oil

1 package firm or extra-firm tofu, pressed and cut into ½-inch dice

1 tablespoon cornstarch

½ teaspoon salt, divided

¼ teaspoon freshly ground black pepper

¼ teaspoon paprika

½ cup cilantro sprigs

½ cup parsley sprigs

½ medium yellow onion, chopped

2 garlic cloves

½ jalapeño, seeded

2 tablespoons extra-virgin olive oil

4 cups cauliflower rice (1 large head)

Grated zest and juice of 1 small lime

1. Preheat the oven to 400°F. Grease a sheet pan or large glass baking dish with the coconut oil.

2. Put the tofu in a medium mixing bowl.

3. Sprinkle with the cornstarch, ¼ teaspoon of salt, and the pepper and paprika. Toss to coat. Transfer to the prepared sheet pan.

4. Transfer the sheet pan to the oven, and bake for 15 minutes. Flip the tofu, and bake for 15 minutes, or until lightly browned on the edges. Remove from the oven.

5. Meanwhile, in a food processor or blender, combine the cilantro, parsley, onion, garlic, and jalapeño. Process, scraping down the side of the bowl as necessary, until the mixture achieves a paste-like consistency. Add water, 1 tablespoon at a time, as needed to get to the desired consistency.

6. In a large skillet, heat the olive oil over medium-high heat.

7. Add the cauliflower rice, and cook, stirring occasionally, for 3 to 4 minutes, or until starting to soften slightly.

8. Stir in the cilantro mixture, and cook, stirring occasionally, for 2 to 3 minutes, or until fragrant. Remove from the heat.

9. Stir in the lime zest and juice and the remaining ¼ teaspoon of salt.

10. Serve the cauliflower rice hot with the tofu on top.

Bioactive ingredients: tofu, parsley, onion, garlic, chile, olive oil, cauliflower

Per Serving: Calories: 209; Total fat: 14g; Saturated fat: 3g; Protein: 12g; Total carbohydrates: 13g; Fiber: 3g; Sugar: 3g; Cholesterol: 0g

→ **VARIATION:** This recipe works well with regular rice, too. Consider using 3 cups cooked brown rice for a high-fiber, nutrient-dense option rather than white. I don't spend a lot of time pressing my tofu to dry it; I prefer to pat it dry and then pop it in the oven, but if you want crispier tofu, take the time to lay paper towels and kitchen towels over slices of tofu and then press using a pot or heavy cutting board (or both) for 20 minutes.

Vegetarian Stuffed Bell Peppers

Gluten-Free, Nut-Free,
Soy-Free, Vegetarian

SERVES 4

PREP TIME: 5 MINUTES / COOK TIME: 40 MINUTES

A classic comfort food, stuffed peppers are a quick, easy, and balanced way to support all five of your body's natural defense systems. Choose whatever color of peppers you enjoy—green, red, orange, or even an heirloom variety that's striped or purple. The amount of filling you use depends on the size of your peppers, and if you have extra left over, you can enjoy it as a snack or lunch the following day on some greens or wrapped in a tortilla.

2 tablespoons extra-virgin olive oil

½ medium yellow onion, diced

2 garlic cloves, minced

1 jalapeño, minced

1½ cups cooked brown rice

1 (15-ounce) can pinto beans, drained and rinsed

1 tomato, diced

1 teaspoon chili powder

1 teaspoon ground cumin

½ teaspoon salt

1 cup shredded Gouda cheese, plus 1 tablespoon

4 bell peppers, tops, seeds, and membranes removed

1. Preheat the oven to 350°F.

2. In a medium skillet, heat the oil over medium heat.

3. Add the onion, and sauté for 3 to 5 minutes, or until translucent.

4. Add the garlic and jalapeño. Cook for 2 to 3 minutes, or until the vegetables start to soften and become fragrant. Remove from the heat.

5. In a large mixing bowl, combine the rice, beans, tomato, chili powder, cumin, salt, and cooked vegetables. Stir until thoroughly mixed.

6. Fold in 1 cup of cheese.

7. Arrange the bell peppers in an 8-by-8-inch baking dish.

8. Carefully spoon the rice and vegetable filling into each one.

9. Sprinkle the bell peppers with the remaining 1 tablespoon of cheese.

10. Transfer the baking dish to the oven, and bake for 30 minutes, or until the cheese has melted and the peppers are fork tender. Remove from the oven.

Per Serving: Calories: 408; Total fat: 17g; Saturated fat: 6g; Protein: 17g; Total carbohydrates: 51g; Fiber: 9g; Sugar: 3g; Cholesterol: 32g

→ **VARIATION:** All beans have beneficial properties, so you can swap in whatever type you prefer or what you have on hand. Navy beans or chickpeas are good substitutions in this recipe. You can further boost the health benefits and flavor of this dish by garnishing it with fresh cilantro.

Bioactive ingredients: olive oil, onion, garlic, chile, brown rice, beans, tomato, cumin, Gouda, bell pepper

Eggplant Lasagna with Quinoa and Spinach

Gluten-Free, Nut-Free, Soy-Free, Vegetarian	**SERVES 8** PREP TIME: 20 MINUTES / COOK TIME: 1 HOUR 5 MINUTES

Traditional lasagna gets a health-promoting lift from antioxidant-packed eggplant "noodles," tomato sauce, and savory ricotta, mozzarella, and Parmigiano-Reggiano cheeses.

1 cup quinoa, rinsed

1¾ cups water

2 medium eggplants, tops and bottoms trimmed off, cut into ¼-inch-thick rounds

¼ cup extra-virgin olive oil

½ teaspoon salt

½ teaspoon freshly ground black pepper

2 cups spinach, coarsely chopped

2 eggs

1 teaspoon dried oregano

1 teaspoon dried basil

1 teaspoon dried parsley

¾ cup ricotta cheese

1 cup grated mozzarella cheese, divided

½ cup shredded Parmigiano-Reggiano cheese, divided

1 (26-ounce) jar marinara sauce

Bioactive ingredients: quinoa, eggplant, olive oil, spinach, oregano, basil, parsley, Parmigiano-Reggiano, tomato

1. Preheat the oven to 375°F. Line 2 sheet pans with parchment paper.

2. In a medium saucepan, combine the quinoa and water. Bring to a boil over high heat.

3. Reduce the heat to medium-low. Cover the saucepan, and cook for 15 minutes, or until the water has been absorbed and the quinoa is fluffy. Remove from the heat. Let rest, covered, for 5 minutes. Transfer to a large bowl.

4. While the quinoa is cooking, arrange the eggplants on the prepared sheet pans.

5. Brush both sides of each piece of eggplant lightly with the oil. Season on one side with the salt and pepper.

6. Transfer the sheet pans to the oven, and roast for 20 minutes, or until the eggplants start to lightly brown. Remove from the oven, leaving the oven on.

7. Stir the spinach into the quinoa. Let rest for an additional 10 minutes so the spinach can soften.

8. In a small mixing bowl, beat the eggs.

9. Whisk the oregano, basil, and parsley into the eggs. Mix the eggs into the softened spinach and quinoa.

10. In a medium mixing bowl, combine the ricotta cheese, ½ cup of mozzarella cheese, and ¼ cup of Parmigiano-Reggiano cheese.

11. Spread 1 cup of marinara sauce evenly in the bottom of a 9-by-13-inch glass baking dish.

12. Place half of the eggplant slices (about 6 pieces) on top of the sauce. Spread half of the quinoa mixture evenly over the eggplant.

13. Spoon half of the ricotta mixture on top of the quinoa mixture so it is spaced evenly around the lasagna.

14. Layer the remaining eggplant on top, then spread about 1 cup of sauce.

15. Cover the sauce with the remaining quinoa mixture, then spoon the remaining ricotta mixture, again evenly spaced, on top of the quinoa.

16. Cover with the remaining sauce. Top with the remaining ½ cup of mozzarella cheese and ¼ cup of Parmigiano-Reggiano cheese. Cover with aluminum foil.

17. Transfer the baking dish to the oven, and bake for 25 minutes. Uncover, then bake for 20 minutes. Remove from the oven.

Per Serving: Calories: 325; Total fat: 18g; Saturated fat: 6g; Protein: 15g; Total carbohydrates: 29g; Fiber: 7g; Sugar: 9g; Cholesterol: 75g

→ **VARIATION:** You can use full- or reduced-fat ricotta, whichever you prefer, but a reduced-fat variety will lower your saturated fat intake. Make sure to rinse your quinoa before cooking, because if you skip that step, the bitter compounds on it can make the dish taste bitter, too.

Garlic Chickpea Bowls with Miso-Tahini Dressing

Dairy-Free, Nut-Free, Vegan	SERVES 4
	PREP TIME: 10 MINUTES / COOK TIME: 50 MINUTES

A simple, balanced bowl is perfect for a busy weekday lunch or dinner and can be altered easily for different tastes within a family or household. Prepare all the healthy ingredients and then set them out for each person to assemble their own bowls, adding more or less dressing or vegetables and adjusting for their favorite toppings. You can use this dressing on other types of salads, as well, or as a dipping sauce for fresh vegetables.

1 cup brown rice

2 cups water

2 tablespoons extra-virgin olive oil

3 garlic cloves, minced, divided

1 (15-ounce) can chickpeas, drained, rinsed, and patted dry

½ teaspoon salt, divided

2 small jalapeños, seeded and chopped

1 (1-inch) piece fresh ginger, grated

1 cup cilantro sprigs

Juice of 1 lime

1 teaspoon maple syrup

⅓ cup tahini

1½ tablespoons miso

4 cups spinach

1 ripe avocado, pitted, peeled, and sliced

1 cup shredded carrot

Bioactive ingredients: brown rice, olive oil, garlic, beans, chile, ginger, tahini, miso, spinach, avocado, carrot

1. In a medium saucepan, combine the rice and water. Bring to a boil.

2. Reduce the heat to low. Cover the saucepan, and simmer for 45 minutes, or until all of the water has been completely absorbed and the rice is fluffy. Remove from the heat.

3. Meanwhile, in a large skillet, heat the oil over medium heat.

4. Add two-thirds of the garlic, and cook for 1 to 2 minutes, or until starting to brown.

5. Add the chickpeas.

6. Increase the heat to medium-high. Cook the chickpeas for 3 minutes. Toss, and continue to cook for 2 minutes more, or until golden brown. Sprinkle with ¼ teaspoon of salt. Remove from the heat.

7. To make the dressing, put the jalapeños, ginger, cilantro, lime juice, maple syrup, tahini, miso, the remaining third of the garlic, and the remaining ¼ teaspoon of salt in a food processor or blender. Pulse until the ingredients are blended. Add water, 1 tablespoon at a time, as needed to make the consistency pourable.

8. Place about ¼ to ⅓ cup of the cooked rice in the bottom of each of 4 bowls, followed by 1 cup of spinach.

9. Arrange the avocado and carrot in sections on top.

10. Drizzle 2 to 3 tablespoons of the dressing over the top of each bowl.

11. Add ¼ cup of the roasted chickpeas on top of each bowl.

Per Serving: Calories: 563; Total fat: 28g; Saturated fat: 4g; Protein: 15g; Total carbohydrates: 68g; Fiber: 14g; Sugar: 8g; Cholesterol: 0g

→ **VARIATION:** If the jalapeño in the dressing is too hot, consider using an Anaheim pepper instead for a milder flavor. You can swap out the cilantro for parsley if desired, and consider using quinoa as a base instead of rice. Swap out the spinach for arugula, kale, or red-leaf lettuce to mix it up.

Farro Energy Bowls with Seasoned Tofu

Nut-Free, Vegetarian

SERVES 4

PREP TIME: 15 MINUTES / COOK TIME: 40 MINUTES

Farro is a high-fiber, nutrient-dense, health-promoting base for this energy bowl. A whole grain, farro is actually a type of wheat. It has a hearty, nutty texture and flavor and is packed full of protein, fiber, magnesium, zinc, and B vitamins. The tofu powers up this energy bowl with antioxidants and protein, and it's topped off with a variety of health-promoting, flavorful vegetables.

1 cup whole-wheat farro

3 cups water

1 teaspoon salt, divided

1 (14-ounce) package firm or extra-firm tofu, drained and pressed

1 tablespoon sesame oil

Juice of 1 small lime

1 tablespoon low-sodium soy sauce

1 ripe avocado, pitted and peeled

⅔ cup nonfat plain Greek yogurt or nondairy yogurt

¼ cup extra-virgin olive oil

Juice of 1 lemon

1 garlic clove

1 teaspoon coconut oil

1½ cups shredded cabbage

1 cup broccoli sprouts or other sprouts or microgreens

2 cups cherry tomatoes, halved

½ cup pumpkin seeds, chopped

Bioactive ingredients: whole-wheat farro, tofu, soy sauce, avocado, yogurt, olive oil, lemon, garlic, cabbage, broccoli sprouts, tomato, pumpkin seed

1. In a medium saucepan, combine the farro, water, and ½ teaspoon of salt. Bring to a boil.

2. Reduce the heat to low. Cover the saucepan, and simmer, stirring occasionally, for 30 to 40 minutes, or until the farro is tender. Remove from the heat. Drain.

3. Meanwhile, cut the tofu crosswise into ½-inch-thick slabs and then cut it again diagonally to create 2 triangles.

4. In a medium bowl, combine the tofu pieces, sesame oil, lime juice, and soy sauce. Let marinate while you make the dressing.

5. Put the avocado, yogurt, olive oil, lemon juice, garlic, and remaining ½ teaspoon of salt in a blender or food processor. Pulse until well blended. Add water, 1 tablespoon at a time, for a total of about 3 tablespoons, or until the dressing is pourable.

6. In a large skillet, heat the coconut oil over medium-high heat.

7. Add the tofu in a single layer, and cook undisturbed for about 3 minutes, or until golden brown.

8. Turn the tofu pieces over, and cook for about 3 minutes, or until browned on the second side. Remove from the heat.

9. Place ¼ to ⅓ cup of the cooked farro in one half of each bowl.

10. Fill the other half of each bowl with the cabbage.

11. Top with the sprouts, tomatoes, and tofu.

12. Drizzle the dressing over the top.

13. Garnish with the pumpkin seeds.

Per Serving: Calories: 664; Total fat: 41g; Saturated fat: 8g; Protein: 24g; Total carbohydrates: 59g; Fiber: 16g; Sugar: 9g; Cholesterol: 5g

→ **VARIATION:** Consider other whole grains to replace the farro, including quinoa, buckwheat, spelt berries, or sorghum if desired. You could add nuts, such as ¼ cup chopped walnuts, almonds, or hazelnuts, in addition to or instead of the pumpkin seeds.

Mushroom, Walnut, and Lentil Loaf

Dairy-Free, Gluten-Free,
Soy-Free, Vegan

SERVES 6

PREP TIME: 15 MINUTES / COOK TIME: 1 HOUR
10 MINUTES, PLUS 30 MINUTES TO COOL

There's no meat needed in this healthy version of a classic meatloaf. Serve this with a side of roasted potatoes and Citrus-Herb Asparagus (page 115), Garlic Bok Choy (page 113), or a fresh, green salad for a balanced meal. Bonus: Lentils are very high in fiber, protein, and minerals.

1 cup green or brown dried
lentils, rinsed

2½ cups vegetable stock

2 tablespoons ground
flaxseed

¼ cup water, plus
1 teaspoon

2 tablespoons extra-virgin
olive oil

½ medium yellow
onion, diced

½ cup mushrooms, diced

1 medium carrot, diced

1 celery stalk, diced

4 garlic cloves, minced

1 teaspoon dried oregano

1 teaspoon dried thyme

1 teaspoon ground cumin

½ teaspoon salt

½ teaspoon freshly ground
black pepper

½ cup walnuts,
finely chopped

¾ cup rolled oats, ground

2 tablespoons tomato paste

1 teaspoon balsamic vinegar

1 tablespoon maple syrup

Bioactive ingredients: lentils, flaxseed, olive oil, onion, mushroom, carrot, celery, garlic, oregano, thyme, cumin, walnut, oats, tomato

1. In a medium saucepan, combine the lentils and stock. Bring to a boil.

2. Reduce the heat to low. Cover the saucepan, and simmer for 30 to 35 minutes, or until the lentils are soft and the stock has mostly been absorbed. Remove from the heat. Drain any excess liquid.

3. To make a flax egg, in a small mixing bowl, mix together the flaxseed and ¼ cup of water. Let sit for at least 10 minutes, or until a gel starts to form.

4. Preheat the oven to 350°F. Line an 8½-by-4½-inch loaf pan with parchment paper.

5. Meanwhile, in a medium skillet, heat the oil over medium heat.

6. Add the onion, mushrooms, carrot, and celery. Sauté for 4 to 6 minutes, or until the onion is translucent and the other vegetables begin to soften.

7. Add the garlic, oregano, thyme, cumin, salt, and pepper. Cook for 3 to 4 minutes, or until the vegetables are soft and the spices are fragrant. Remove from the heat.

8. Put the lentils, flax egg, walnuts, and oats in a food processor. Pulse until the mixture has a paste-like texture. Transfer to a large mixing bowl.

9. Stir in the cooked vegetables. Transfer to the prepared loaf pan.

10. In a small bowl, mix together the tomato paste, vinegar, maple syrup, and remaining 1 teaspoon of water to create a glaze.

11. Spread the glaze on top of the loaf.

12. Transfer the loaf pan to the oven, and bake for 30 minutes, or until the edges of the loaf darken. Remove from the oven. Let the loaf cool in the pan for 15 minutes, then transfer the loaf with the parchment paper to a cooling rack, and let cool for another 15 minutes.

Per Serving: Calories: 318; Total fat: 13g; Saturated fat: 2g; Protein: 13g; Total carbohydrates: 39g; Fiber: 7g; Sugar: 5g; Cholesterol: 0g

→ **VARIATION:** This recipe is vegan, but if you want to substitute an egg for the flax egg, then simply skip step 3, and add a whole egg during step 8. If you are cooking for picky eaters, you can use the food processor to blend the vegetable mixture into the loaf.

Chilled Soba with Sesame Tempeh

Dairy-Free, Nut-Free, Vegetarian	SERVES 4
	PREP TIME: 20 MINUTES / COOK TIME: 15 MINUTES

Soba is typically made out of buckwheat, a whole grain. It cooks quickly and makes great leftovers to serve alongside other ingredients that help boost health by offering a variety of vitamins, minerals, and antioxidants. Tempeh is a microbiome-boosting plant-based protein option that's firmer than tofu and therefore a great substitution for anyone who wants a tofu alternative while keeping all the health benefits of this superfood. If you're trying to eat less meat, tempeh could be a great option for you.

5 tablespoons low-sodium soy sauce, divided

5 tablespoons sesame oil, divided

½ teaspoon honey, plus 1 tablespoon

1 garlic clove, minced

1 (½-inch) piece fresh ginger, grated

1 (8-ounce) package tempeh, cut into ¼-inch-thick slices

12 ounces buckwheat soba

2 tablespoons rice vinegar

Grated zest and juice of 1 lime

2 tablespoons tahini

1 medium cucumber, halved lengthwise, seeded, then cut into thin half-moons

1 red bell pepper, seeded and thinly sliced

⅓ cup thinly sliced scallions, green and white parts

½ cup sesame seeds

Bioactive ingredients: soy sauce, garlic, ginger, tempeh, buckwheat, tahini, bell pepper, onion, sesame seed

1. To make the marinade, in a small mixing bowl, whisk together 2 tablespoons of soy sauce, 1 tablespoon of oil, ½ teaspoon of honey, and the garlic and ginger.

2. Put the tempeh in an 8-by-8-inch glass baking dish.

3. Pour the marinade on top.

4. While the tempeh is soaking in the marinade, bring a large pot of water to a boil over high heat.

5. Add the soba, and cook for 5 minutes. Remove from the heat. Drain immediately, then rinse with cold water; drain again thoroughly. Transfer to a large mixing bowl.

6. Add 2 tablespoons of oil, and toss. Chill in the refrigerator.

7. Preheat the oven to 375°F. Line a sheet pan with parchment paper or a silicone liner.

8. To make the dressing, in a small mixing bowl, whisk together the vinegar, lime zest and juice, tahini, and remaining 3 tablespoons of soy sauce, 1 tablespoon of honey, and 2 tablespoons of oil. If needed, add water, 1 tablespoon at a time, to achieve your desired consistency and volume. (If the honey and tahini aren't soft enough to whisk, you can also put all of these ingredients in a blender, and blend until smooth.)

9. Pour the tempeh onto the prepared sheet pan, and scrape any remaining marinade out of the bowl and on top of the tempeh.

10. Transfer the sheet pan to the oven, and bake, flipping the tempeh halfway through, for 15 minutes, or until lightly browned. Remove from the oven.

11. While the tempeh is baking, pour the dressing over the soba, and toss gently to coat.

12. Stir in the cucumber, bell pepper, and scallions, making sure they are well distributed throughout. Store the soba in the refrigerator until ready to serve.

13. Serve the soba topped with the tempeh and sesame seeds.

Per Serving: Calories: 753; Total fat: 39g; Saturated fat: 6g; Protein: 31g; Total carbohydrates: 81g; Fiber: 4g; Sugar: 5g; Cholesterol: 0g

→ **VARIATION:** To make this a vegan dish, simply replace the honey with maple syrup or agave syrup. You can use ¼ cup chopped chives in place of the scallions. For a bolder flavor, lightly toast your sesame seeds in a dry pan over medium-low heat for about 3 to 4 minutes.

Red Lentil Curry with Cauliflower

Dairy-Free, Gluten-Free,
Nut-Free, Soy-Free, Vegan

SERVES 6

PREP TIME: 10 MINUTES / COOK TIME: 45 MINUTES

High-fiber red lentils combine with vibrant, immune-boosting herbs and spices to create a fragrant stew to serve over rice. Lentils contain both soluble and insoluble fiber to support the gut microbiome and help lower cholesterol levels. They also keep you feeling full and satisfied long after your meal. This dish makes excellent leftovers to refrigerate or freeze for later meals.

1 cup brown rice

4½ cups water, divided

2 tablespoons extra-virgin olive oil

½ yellow onion, finely chopped

1 tablespoon grated fresh ginger

2 garlic cloves, minced

1 teaspoon ground cumin

½ teaspoon ground coriander

1 teaspoon grated fresh turmeric root or ½ teaspoon turmeric

1 teaspoon salt

1½ cups dried red lentils

1 (13½-ounce) can light coconut milk

1 small head cauliflower, chopped into florets

1 cup cilantro leaves

1. In a medium saucepan, combine the rice and 2 cups of water. Bring to a boil over high heat.

2. Reduce the heat to low. Cover the saucepan, and simmer for 45 minutes, or until the water has been completely absorbed and the rice is fluffy. Remove from the heat.

3. Meanwhile, in a large stockpot, heat the oil over medium heat.

4. Add the onion, and cook for about 5 minutes, or until soft and translucent.

5. Add the ginger and garlic. Cook, stirring constantly, for 1 minute.

6. Add the cumin, coriander, turmeric, and salt. Cook, stirring, for 1 minute.

7. Add the remaining 2½ cups of water, the lentils, and the coconut milk. Stir well to combine.

8. Reduce the heat to medium-low. Cover the saucepan, and cook for 10 minutes.

9. Add the cauliflower, and cook for 7 to 10 minutes, or until the cauliflower is easily pierced using a fork and the lentils are soft. Remove from the heat.

10. Serve the lentil curry over the rice, garnished with the cilantro.

Per Serving: Calories: 396; Total fat: 12g; Saturated fat: 5g; Protein: 15g; Total carbohydrates: 58g; Fiber: 8g; Sugar: 2g; Cholesterol: 0g

→ **VARIATION:** You can swap out the cauliflower and add 1 cup chopped carrots instead. If you do so, reduce the cooking time in step 9 to 5 to 6 minutes. If you want to experiment with romanesco instead of regular cauliflower, the cooking time and portion will be the same, but you'll get a slightly firmer texture and milder flavor.

Bioactive ingredients: brown rice, olive oil, onion, ginger, garlic, cumin, turmeric, lentils, cauliflower

Penne with Pesto and Antipasti

Vegetarian	**SERVES 6**
	PREP TIME: 10 MINUTES / COOK TIME: 15 MINUTES

Give a simple pasta dish even more disease-fighting nutrition by making your own pesto with protein from silken tofu. Serve this with roasted tempeh or chicken, a simple side salad, and sourdough bread (see page 140) with roasted garlic for even more immune-boosting potential.

12 ounces penne, preferably whole-wheat or bean pasta

2 cups packed fresh basil leaves

1 tablespoon dried oregano

⅓ cup pine nuts, toasted

4 garlic cloves, minced

¼ cup extra-virgin olive oil

2 teaspoons freshly squeezed lemon juice

1 teaspoon salt

6 ounces (½ package) extra-firm silken tofu, drained

1 ounce Parmigiano-Reggiano cheese, finely grated (about ½ cup)

1 cup Kalamata olives, pitted and chopped

1 (15-ounce) can artichoke hearts, drained and quartered

½ cup chopped fresh parsley

Bioactive ingredients: basil, oregano, pine nut, garlic, olive oil, lemon, tofu, Parmigiano-Reggiano, artichoke, parsley

1. Fill a large stockpot two-thirds full of water. Bring to a boil over high heat. Add the penne, and cook according to the package instructions (usually 9 to 12 minutes). Remove from the heat. Drain, and return to the pot.

2. Meanwhile, to make the pesto, in a food processor or blender, combine the basil, oregano, pine nuts, garlic, oil, lemon juice, salt, and tofu. Puree until completely smooth.

3. Add the pesto to the pot. Cook over medium heat, stirring until coated, for about 1 minute. Remove from the heat.

4. Stir in the cheese, olives, and artichoke hearts.

5. Garnish with the parsley, and serve hot or cold.

Per Serving: Calories: 437; Total fat: 21g; Saturated fat: 3g; Protein: 16g; Total carbohydrates: 55g; Fiber: 11g; Sugar: 1g; Cholesterol: 4g

→ **VARIATION:** Replace the cheese with 1 tablespoon nutritional yeast for a vegan version.

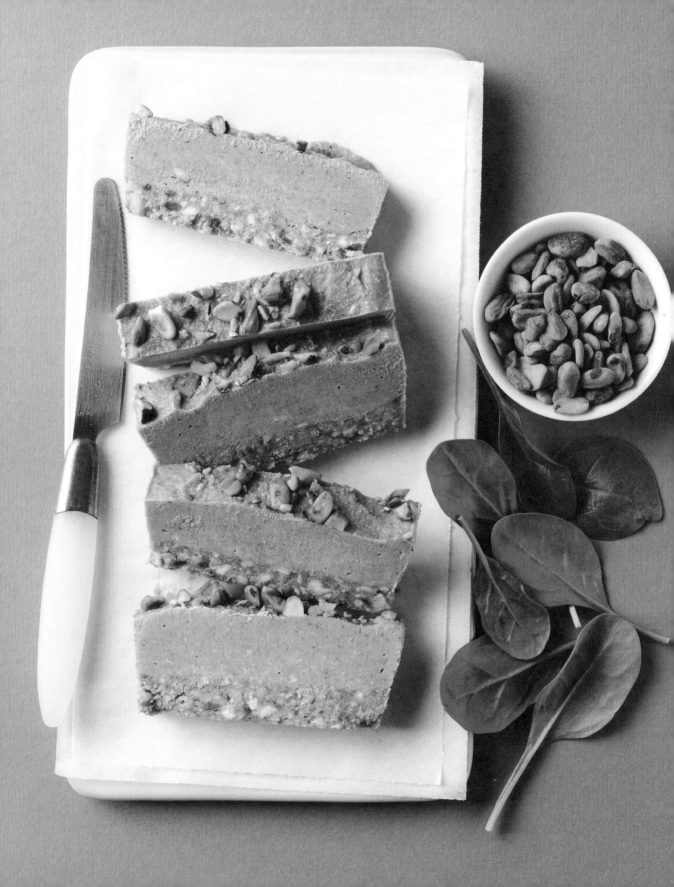

CHAPTER 8

Desserts and Baking

There's no reason why baked goods and sweet treats can't be made in a way that helps you meet your health goals. Health-promoting fruits, vegetables, nuts, seeds, and even beans can be easily added into delicious recipes, helping support your immune system, microbiome, DNA health, and stem cells, and even helping manage the angiogenesis process. Whether you're making your own sourdough, serving up some black bean brownies, or making a dessert out of seasonal fruit and whole grains, these recipes can help show you that the balance of flavor and health really does exist.

Sourdough Starter

Dairy-Free, Nut-Free,
Soy-Free, Vegan

**MAKES 1½ CUPS
SOURDOUGH STARTER**

PREP TIME: 5-DAY PROCESS

Sourdough has become more popular than ever, and baking at home is a wonderful way to support your health and feel connected to your food. If you don't already have a sourdough starter, there are a few ways to get one. You can make one with this recipe, get one from a friend, or order one online. Some people even have sourdough starters that have been passed down through generations (and they're often willing to share). Keep in mind that making a starter takes about five days with a small task every day.

1 cup whole-wheat flour

2 to 2½ cups filtered warm
(not hot) water, divided

3 to 4 cups bread
flour, divided

MAKE THE INITIAL STARTER (DAY 1)

1. In a 2-quart glass measuring cup, jar, or large bowl, combine the whole-wheat flour and ½ cup of water. Mix until a smooth batter forms. It should resemble a loose, wet dough. Cover the container with a clean, tightly knit kitchen towel, flour sack towel, or plastic wrap. Secure with a rubber band.

2. Store the container somewhere with a consistent room temperature of 70°F to 75°F that's not in direct sunlight for 24 hours. Consider the top of your refrigerator or a counter away from a window.

FEED THE STARTER (DAYS 2 THROUGH 4)

3. Each day you check the starter, it should have bubbles on top, ideally more each day, eventually appearing frothy. It may develop a slightly sour or yeasty odor.

4. Each day, at the same time of day, stir the mixture, then discard all but ½ cup of the starter, then add 1 cup of bread flour and ½ cup of water to the existing starter bowl. Mix until it forms the loose, wet dough again. Cover, secure, and store the container in the same way as you did on day 1.

STARTER IS READY TO USE (DAY 5 AND BEYOND)

5. Between days 4 and 5, the volume of starter should about double. It will look quite bubbly and smell slightly sour. If it doesn't seem as active as the description or there aren't many bubbles, you may need to let it go one more day, feeding it with the flour and water mixture as on days 2, 3, and 4. One way to know whether it's done is to take 1 teaspoon of the starter from the top of the mixture and drop it in a glass full of water. If it floats, then it's ready, and if it doesn't float, then you should go through another cycle of feeding and resting. If the starter is very bubbly and sour-smelling and floats when you drop a teaspoon of it in water, you can start using it to bake with on day 5.

6. To maintain the starter over time, on day 5, use it in the Basic, No-Knead Sourdough Loaf (page 140) or Fluffy Sourdough Pancakes (page 45), or discard half of it, and then feed it once more like you have been doing on days 2 through 4.

7. You can now store your starter in the refrigerator in a glass jar or bowl, covered tightly with plastic wrap. Pour out any liquid that develops on the top. From now on you only need to feed the starter once per week. When you feed it, remember to discard all but ½ cup, then stir in 1 cup bread flour and ½ cup water. (You can use what you need during the week so long as the base amount does not fall below ½ cup.)

Per Serving (¼ cup): Calories: 108; Total fat: 1g; Saturated fat: 0g; Protein: 4g; Total carbohydrates: 23g; Fiber: 2g; Sugar: 0g; Cholesterol: 0g

→ **VARIATION:** There are a lot of variables when it comes to making a starter: what kind of flour you use, what kind of water, the temperature in your house, and the type and amount of wild yeast present in your environment. With so many unknowns, you may need to troubleshoot based on your unique circumstances.

Basic, No-Knead Sourdough Loaf

Dairy-Free, Nut-Free,
Soy-Free, Vegan

SERVES 8

PREP TIME: 12 HOURS / COOK TIME: 35 MINUTES

It's surprisingly easy to make your own fresh sourdough at home, especially when you use a simple, no-knead recipe. Work the bread around your own schedule, either starting the process in the evening at 4 p.m. by making your dough, then baking it in the morning, or making the dough at 8 a.m. and baking it that evening. This is designed to be a very basic, relatively quick version, but there are much more complex options if you enjoy that type of bread-making experience. If you want to get really creative, you can use the sourdough starter recipe in this book (see page 138), or you can use a starter that you've purchased or received from a friend or family member.

2 tablespoons
   sourdough starter

1 cup warm (not hot) water

3 cups bread flour, plus
   more for dusting

1 teaspoon salt

1 tablespoon extra-virgin
   olive oil, divided

Bioactive ingredient:
sourdough bread

1. In a small mixing bowl, combine the starter and water.

2. In a large mixing bowl, combine the flour and salt.

3. Pour the wet ingredients into the dry ingredients. Using a wooden spoon, mix until a dry dough forms.

4. Cover the dough with a clean kitchen cloth or paper towel. Let sit for 20 minutes in a warm, non-drafty place in your kitchen.

5. Using your hands, stretch the dough in the bowl, pulling it softly apart while you stretch it and then fold it in half 4 times, turning 90 degrees each time and stretching the dough again before each fold.

6. Lift the dough from the bowl, and quickly grease the bowl with ½ tablespoon of oil. Return the dough to the bowl.

7. Cover the dough. Let rest for 20 minutes, then stretch and fold once more exactly like you did in step 5.

8. Grease the bowl with the remaining ½ tablespoon of oil. Cover with a cloth or paper towel. Let rest on the kitchen counter overnight, or 8 to 12 hours, until about doubled in size.

9. In the last 30 minutes of rising time, when you're ready to bake the bread, preheat the oven to 500°F. Put a Dutch oven or bread baker in the oven so it heats up. Lightly flour a work surface.

10. Place the dough on the prepared surface. Stretch, fold, and turn 90 degrees twice more, like you did in steps 5 and 7. On your final fold, make sure that the dough forms into a ball, then place it, seam-side down, on a piece of parchment paper large enough to put in your heated Dutch oven or bread baker.

11. Once the oven is heated, use the parchment paper to lift your dough and put it in the hot Dutch oven or bread baker.

12. Sprinkle the top of the dough lightly with flour, and rub it in lightly with your hands. Using a sharp knife, score the bread on top, making a small *x*.

13. Bake the loaf for 30 to 35 minutes, or until the top is golden brown. If the top is browning early, consider reducing the oven temperature to 450°F for the remainder of the baking time. Remove from the oven. Let the bread cool in the Dutch oven for 5 minutes before transferring to a wire rack to cool completely.

Per Serving: Calories: 186; Total fat: 2g; Saturated fat: 0g; Protein: 5g; Total carbohydrates: 36g; Fiber: 1g; Sugar: 0g; Cholesterol: 0g

→ **VARIATION:** There are whole-wheat adaptations that help add fiber and nutrients, but using all-purpose bread flour creates a lighter sourdough product that most people are familiar with.

Cherry-Chocolate Dessert Smoothie

Dairy-Free, Gluten-Free, Vegan

SERVES 2

PREP TIME: 5 MINUTES

Smoothies aren't just for breakfast! Try a decadent, rich chocolate version that's naturally sweetened with health-promoting fruit and complemented with smooth almond butter for heart-healthy fat. There's a secret ingredient in this recipe: spinach! It provides even more immune support that won't change the flavor of your dessert at all. If you've got a sweet tooth, this can be a healthy and delicious replacement for other options that are high in added sugar and saturated fat.

3 cups unsweetened
   soy milk

1 cup frozen cherries

1 frozen banana

½ cup baby spinach

1 tablespoon unsweetened
   cocoa powder

2 tablespoons
   almond butter

Bioactive ingredients: soy milk, cherry, spinach, cocoa, almond

Put the soy milk, cherries, banana, spinach, cocoa powder, and almond butter in a blender. Pulse until smooth.

Per Serving: Calories: 303; Total fat: 13g; Saturated fat: 1g; Protein: 14g; Total carbohydrates: 40g; Fiber: 7g; Sugar: 25g; Cholesterol: 0g

→ **VARIATION:** Frozen cherries and banana help with the thick texture and cool temperature of the smoothie. If you want to use fresh varieties, you can add ½ cup ice in addition to the other ingredients. Add more milk for a thinner smoothie or less for a thicker one. If you are looking for more protein, add a protein powder of your choice, or consider peanut powder. For added sweetness, add a pitted medjool date.

Blackberry Oat Crisp with Lemon Zest

Nut-Free, Soy-Free, Vegetarian

SERVES 8

PREP TIME: 10 MINUTES / COOK TIME: 40 MINUTES

Fresh blackberries taste great in this easy and healthy crisp, but if they're not in season, you can absolutely use frozen berries. Studies show that they maintain their nutrition as much as (or more than) fresh (Li et al. 2017).

1 teaspoon coconut oil

4 cups fresh or frozen blackberries

¼ cup granulated sugar

½ cup rolled oats

¼ cup dairy or nondairy butter, at room temperature

⅓ cup whole-wheat flour

2 tablespoons brown sugar

¼ teaspoon ground cinnamon

¼ teaspoon ground nutmeg

¼ teaspoon ground ginger

½ teaspoon grated lemon zest

Bioactive ingredients: blackberry, oats, whole-wheat flour, cinnamon, ginger, lemon

1. Preheat the oven to 350°F. Grease an 8-by-8-inch baking dish with the oil.

2. In a medium mixing bowl, combine the berries and granulated sugar. Gently fold to coat.

3. In another medium mixing bowl, combine the oats, butter, flour, brown sugar, cinnamon, nutmeg, ginger, and lemon zest. Using a wooden spoon or your fingertips, work the ingredients together until the mixture is crumbly.

4. Pour the berries into the prepared baking dish, scraping any additional sugar out of the bowl and on top of the berries.

5. Spread the oat mixture evenly on top of the berries.

6. Transfer the baking dish to the oven, and bake for 35 to 40 minutes, or until the crisp is lightly browned and the berries are bubbling and soft. Remove from the oven. Set on a cooling rack, and let cool slightly. Serve warm.

Per Serving: Calories: 168; Total fat: 7g; Saturated fat: 4g; Protein: 3g; Total carbohydrates: 24g; Fiber: 5g; Sugar: 12g; Cholesterol: 15g

Spiced Carrot and Nut Muffins

Dairy-Free, Vegetarian

SERVES 12

PREP TIME: 10 MINUTES / COOK TIME: 20 MINUTES

Freshly grated carrot gives these easy muffins a boost of fiber, vitamins, minerals, and antioxidants. Getting vegetables into baked goods is easy to do and adds to the flavor and texture when you combine them with a little sweetness and some familiar spices, like cinnamon and ginger, for complexity.

2 cups grated fresh carrots (about 2 carrots)

1 cup whole-wheat flour

1 cup all-purpose flour

1 teaspoon baking powder

1 teaspoon baking soda

1 teaspoon ground cinnamon

½ teaspoon ground ginger

½ teaspoon salt

2 eggs

½ cup maple syrup

½ cup unsweetened soy milk

¼ cup grapeseed oil or avocado oil

1 teaspoon pure vanilla extract

½ cup chopped macadamia nuts

Bioactive ingredients: carrot, whole-wheat flour, cinnamon, ginger, soy milk, macadamia nut

1. Preheat the oven to 375°F. Line a 12-cup muffin tin with paper liners or silicone liners.

2. Press the carrots gently between paper towels to remove excess moisture.

3. In a large mixing bowl, whisk together the whole-wheat flour, all-purpose flour, baking powder, baking soda, cinnamon, ginger, and salt.

4. In a medium mixing bowl, whisk together the eggs, maple syrup, soy milk, oil, and vanilla.

5. Pour the wet mixture into the dry mixture. Stir to combine.

6. Gently fold in the carrots and nuts until just incorporated.

7. Portion the batter evenly into the prepared muffin tin.

8. Transfer the muffin tin to the oven, and bake for 18 to 20 minutes, or until the muffins are golden brown and firm when you press on the top. Remove from the oven.

Per Serving: Calories: 213; Total fat: 10g; Saturated fat: 1g; Protein: 4g; Total carbohydrates: 28g; Fiber: 3g; Sugar: 10g; Cholesterol: 31g

Cinnamon-Pecan Baked Apples

Gluten-Free, Soy-Free, Vegetarian

SERVES 4

PREP TIME: 15 MINUTES / COOK TIME: 50 MINUTES

Baked apples are a year-round dessert that is simple to prepare and makes your house smell warm and delicious. Consider serving these with vanilla yogurt for a protein-packed breakfast, snack, or dessert.

¼ teaspoon ground cinnamon

¼ teaspoon ground ginger

⅛ teaspoon ground nutmeg

⅛ teaspoon ground cloves

½ cup chopped pecans

¼ cup rolled oats

1 tablespoon maple syrup

1 tablespoon butter or nondairy butter, cut into small pieces

2 medium apples

½ cup water

Bioactive ingredients: cinnamon, ginger, pecan, oats, apple

1. Preheat the oven to 375°F.

2. In a small mixing bowl, mix together the cinnamon, ginger, nutmeg, and cloves.

3. Add the pecans, oats, and maple syrup. Stir to coat the pecans evenly. Add the butter, and toss to coat.

4. Using a paring knife, remove the core of the apples, leaving about ¼ inch at the bottom to hold the filling. Carve the opening about an inch wide so there's plenty of room for the filling.

5. Scoop the pecan filling into each of the apples.

6. Arrange the apples in an 8-by-8-inch glass baking dish. Pour the water into the bottom of the dish to protect the apples from burning.

7. Transfer the baking dish to the oven, and bake for 40 to 50 minutes, or until the apples are soft. Remove from the oven.

Per Serving: Calories: 212; Total fat: 13g; Saturated fat: 3g; Protein: 3g; Total carbohydrates: 23g; Fiber: 5g; Sugar: 13g; Cholesterol: 8g

→ **VARIATION:** Instead of mixing your own spices, you can always use 2 teaspoons of an already prepared pumpkin spice blend.

Classic Black Bean Brownies

Vegetarian

SERVES 9

PREP TIME: 15 MINUTES / COOK TIME:
30 MINUTES, PLUS 15 MINUTES TO COOL

No one would ever be able to tell that there's a superfood ingredient in these brownies: black beans. They incorporate perfectly, adding to the nutrition as well as the moist texture of this recipe. Beans are antiangiogenic and promote a healthy microbiome because they're so high in fiber. Once you try black beans in brownies, you'll never want to make them without!

1 teaspoon coconut oil

⅓ cup all-purpose flour

½ teaspoon baking powder

½ teaspoon salt

¾ cup canned black beans, drained and rinsed

½ cup extra-virgin olive oil

2 eggs

½ cup granulated sugar

¼ cup unsweetened cocoa powder

1 teaspoon pure vanilla extract

½ cup chocolate chips

½ cup walnuts, chopped

¼ cup powdered sugar, for dusting

Bioactive ingredients: beans, olive oil, cocoa, walnut

1. Preheat the oven to 350°F. Grease a 9-by-9-inch baking pan with the coconut oil.

2. In a small bowl, whisk together the flour, baking powder, and salt.

3. In a blender or food processor, combine the beans and olive oil. Puree until blended and pourable.

4. To make the batter, in a stand mixer, combine the bean mixture, eggs, granulated sugar, cocoa powder, and vanilla. Mix on medium-high speed for 15 to 30 seconds, or until smooth.

5. Add the flour mixture. Mix for 15 to 30 seconds, or until incorporated.

6. Add the chocolate chips and walnuts. Mix for 10 to 15 seconds, or until incorporated. Turn off the mixer.

7. Pour the batter into the prepared pan.

8. Transfer the baking pan to the oven, and bake for about 30 minutes, or until the surface is matte around the edges and still shiny in the middle. Remove from the oven. Let the brownies cool for at least 15 minutes before cutting and removing from the pan.

9. Dust with the powdered sugar before serving.

Per Serving: Calories: 315; Total fat: 22g; Saturated fat: 5g; Protein: 5g; Total carbohydrates: 27g; Fiber: 3g; Sugar: 16g; Cholesterol: 42g

→ **VARIATION:** You can leave out the walnuts if desired, though you'll lose the health benefits associated with them. Consider using the same amount of chopped macadamia nuts, hazelnuts, or almonds for a different flavor.

Scallion-Herb Whole-Wheat Scones

Nut-Free

SERVES 8

PREP TIME: 15 MINUTES / COOK TIME: 25 MINUTES

Think beyond sweet berry scones to create an herbal, savory option instead. Rich cheese offers some health benefits, especially to the gut microbiome, and adds an even more complex flavor. Packed full of fresh, flavorful herbs, these scones are perfect for breakfast, brunch, or even a snack.

1½ cups whole-wheat pastry flour

½ cup all-purpose flour, plus 2 tablespoons

1 tablespoon baking powder

¾ teaspoon salt

3 tablespoons cold dairy or nondairy butter, coarsely chopped

1 cup shredded traditional or smoked Gouda, Edam, or Jarlsberg cheese

½ cup minced scallions, green and white parts

½ tablespoon chopped fresh thyme leaves

½ tablespoon minced fresh sage leaves

1 cup unsweetened soy milk

2 tablespoons olive oil

½ teaspoon chopped fresh rosemary leaves

Bioactive ingredients: whole-wheat flour, Gouda, onion, thyme, sage, soy milk, olive oil, rosemary

1. Preheat the oven to 425°F. Line a sheet pan with parchment paper.

2. In a large mixing bowl, mix together the pastry flour, ½ cup of all-purpose flour, the baking powder, and the salt.

3. Add the butter, and using a pastry cutter or 2 knives, incorporate it into the flour until it resembles crumbs or small peas.

4. Add the cheese, scallions, thyme, and sage. Stir until evenly distributed.

5. Pour in the soy milk, and stir just until a dough is formed.

6. Dust a clean work surface with the remaining 2 tablespoons of all-purpose flour.

7. Transfer the dough to the prepared surface. Shape into a large round disk, flattening gently using your palms until about 2 inches thick.

8. Using a butter knife, cut the dough into 8 even triangles.

9. Arrange the triangles of dough about 1 inch apart on the prepared sheet pan.

10. Brush each piece of dough with the oil.

11. Sprinkle a bit of rosemary on top of each.

12. Transfer the sheet pan to the oven, and bake for 18 to 22 minutes, or until the scones are golden brown and cooked through. Remove from the oven. Let cool for 3 to 5 minutes.

Per Serving: Calories: 244; Total fat: 13g; Saturated fat: 6g; Protein: 8g; Total carbohydrates: 26g; Fiber: 3g; Sugar: 2g; Cholesterol: 28g

→ **VARIATION:** Swap out the scallions for ⅓ cup minced chives or ½ cup diced yellow onion instead. You can substitute oregano, or even basil, for the thyme and sage depending on the flavor profile you want in your scone.

Pistachio Bars

| Dairy-Free, Vegan | **SERVES 9** |
| | PREP TIME: 25 MINUTES, PLUS 4 TO 5 HOURS TO FREEZE |

This simple, no-bake dessert or snack is packed full of fiber, protein, and antioxidants that support your health. You'll need a food processor and a loaf pan for this quick recipe; no oven or stovetop is required. The spinach adds a fun green color to complement the pistachios; plus, it's a great way to get more vegetables into your sweet treats. Make sure to allow enough time for this recipe to freeze fully and set up.

⅔ cup pitted dates
(6 to 9 medium dates)

1 cup unsalted cashews

1 cup shelled raw pistachios,
plus 2 tablespoons

2 tablespoons
whole-wheat flour

¼ teaspoon salt

⅓ cup maple syrup

¾ cup unsweetened
soy milk

½ teaspoon pure
vanilla extract

¼ cup spinach

Bioactive ingredients: cashew, pistachio, whole-wheat flour, soy milk, spinach

1. Line an 8½-by-4½-inch loaf pan with parchment paper.

2. Set up 3 small bowls: put the dates in the first, the cashews in the second, and 1 cup of pistachios in the third. Add just enough warm water to cover the ingredient in each bowl. Soak for 15 minutes.

3. Put the dates, ½ cup of the cashews, the flour, and the salt in a food processor. Pulse until the dough just begins to form a ball.

4. Transfer the dough to the prepared loaf pan. Press it down evenly using your fingertips. Store in the freezer while you make the filling.

5. In the food processor, combine the soaked pistachios, maple syrup, soy milk, vanilla, spinach, and remaining ½ cup of the cashews. Blend until smooth and well combined.

6. Remove the loaf pan from the freezer. Pour the filling on top.

7. Chop the remaining 2 tablespoons of pistachios. Sprinkle over the filling.

8. Cover the pan. Freeze for 4 to 5 hours, or until fully set.

9. Gently pull the parchment paper out of the pan to release the loaf, then cut into ½-inch-thick slices. If the parchment is sticking, dip the pan in warm water for 60 seconds to help loosen. Serve the bars, or store covered in the freezer for up to 1 week.

Per Serving: Calories: 243; Total fat: 14g; Saturated fat: 2g; Protein: 6g; Total carbohydrates: 27g; Fiber: 3g; Sugar: 17g; Cholesterol: 0g

→ **VARIATION:** For a gluten-free option, substitute oat or almond flour for the wheat flour. You could use 2 teaspoons matcha green tea powder instead of or in addition to the spinach for a boost of all five defense systems.

Raspberry, Ginger, and Hazelnut Chia Pudding

Dairy-Free, Gluten-Free, Vegetarian

SERVES 4

PREP TIME: 5 MINUTES, PLUS 8 HOURS TO SET

Chia seed pudding is a high-fiber, nutrient-dense, health-promoting, and delicious way to enjoy pudding. Chia seeds are packed with omega-3 fatty acids and protein, and although they're dry and crunchy on their own, once you add a liquid, they become mucilaginous and form a gel perfect for recipes like this one. Enjoy this pudding as a simple breakfast, snack, or dessert.

½ cup chia seeds

2 cups unsweetened soy milk

1 teaspoon ground ginger

1 teaspoon pure vanilla extract

2 teaspoons honey

½ cup chopped hazelnuts

1 cup fresh or frozen red or black raspberries

Bioactive ingredients: chia seed, soy milk, ginger, hazelnut, raspberry

1. In a medium mixing bowl, whisk together the chia seeds, soy milk, ginger, vanilla, and honey. Cover with a lid or plastic wrap. Let set for 6 to 8 hours or overnight in the refrigerator, stirring well after 1 to 3 hours to incorporate any of the seeds that have settled to the bottom or are stuck to the side.

2. Divide the pudding among 4 small serving bowls or jars.

3. Top with the hazelnuts and raspberries. Serve chilled.

Per Serving: Calories: 325; Total fat: 20g; Saturated fat: 2g; Protein: 11g; Total carbohydrates: 29g; Fiber: 14g; Sugar: 10g; Cholesterol: 0g

→ **VARIATION:** You may need to add more milk if you prefer a thinner pudding or if yours is too thick and not a pudding texture. You could use the same amount of walnuts, almonds, pecans, or peanuts instead of hazelnuts and the same amount of other fruit, such as strawberries, blackberries, or chopped cherries, instead of the raspberries. Use maple syrup instead of honey for a vegan recipe.

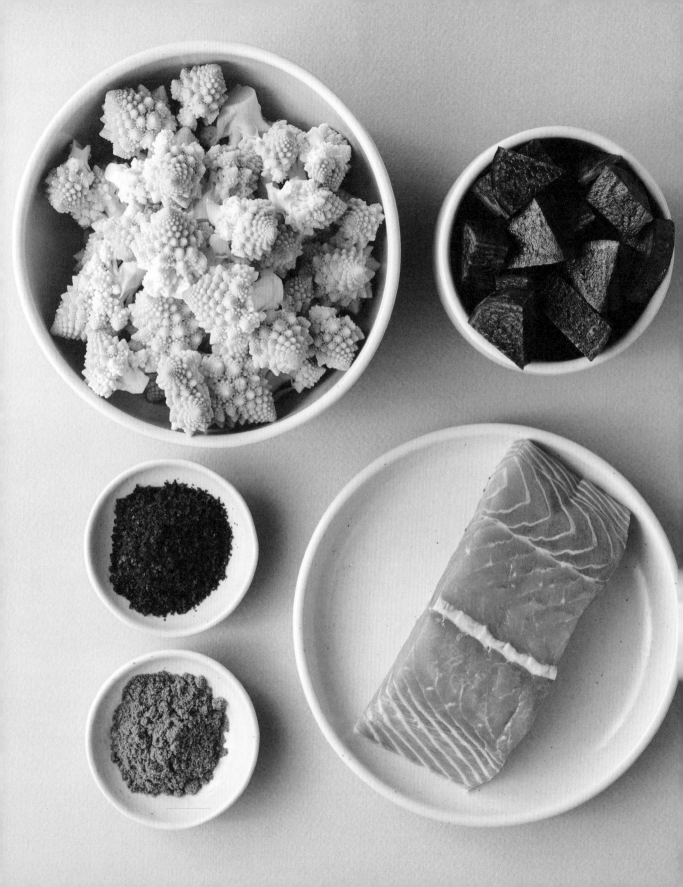

MEASUREMENT CONVERSIONS

VOLUME EQUIVALENTS	U.S. STANDARD	U.S. STANDARD (OUNCES)	METRIC (APPROXIMATE)
LIQUID	2 tablespoons	1 fl. oz.	30 mL
	¼ cup	2 fl. oz.	60 mL
	½ cup	4 fl. oz.	120 mL
	1 cup	8 fl. oz.	240 mL
	1½ cups	12 fl. oz.	355 mL
	2 cups or 1 pint	16 fl. oz.	475 mL
	4 cups or 1 quart	32 fl. oz.	1 L
	1 gallon	128 fl. oz.	4 L
DRY	⅛ teaspoon		0.5 mL
	¼ teaspoon		1 mL
	½ teaspoon		2 mL
	¾ teaspoon		4 mL
	1 teaspoon		5 mL
	1 tablespoon		15 mL
	¼ cup		59 mL
	⅓ cup		79 mL
	½ cup		118 mL
	⅔ cup		156 mL
	¾ cup		177 mL
	1 cup		235 mL
	2 cups or 1 pint		475 mL
	3 cups		700 mL
	4 cups or 1 quart		1 L
	½ gallon		2 L
	1 gallon		4 L

OVEN TEMPERATURES

FAHRENHEIT	CELSIUS (APPROXIMATE)
250°F	120°C
300°F	150°C
325°F	165°C
350°F	180°C
375°F	190°C
400°F	200°C
425°F	220°C
450°F	230°C

WEIGHT EQUIVALENTS

U.S. STANDARD	METRIC (APPROXIMATE)
½ ounce	15 g
1 ounce	30 g
2 ounces	60 g
4 ounces	115 g
8 ounces	225 g
12 ounces	340 g
16 ounces or 1 pound	455 g

REFERENCES

Abbasi, Jennifer. "TMAO and Heart Disease: The New Red Meat Risk?" *Journal of the American Medical Association* 321, no. 22 (June 2019): 2149–51. doi.org/10.1001/jama.2019.3910.

Abbaszadeh, Hassan, Bijan Keikhaei, and Sayeh Mottaghi. "A Review of Molecular Mechanisms Involved in Anticancer and Antiangiogenic Effects of Natural Polyphenolic Compounds." *Phytotherapy Research* 33, no. 8 (August 2019): 2002–14. doi.org/10.1002/ptr.6403.

Abdelhamid, Asmaa S., Tracey J. Brown, Julii S. Brainard, Priti Biswas, Gabrielle C. Thorpe, Helen J. Moore, Katherine H.O. Deane, et al. "Omega-3 Fatty Acids for the Primary and Secondary Prevention of Cardiovascular Disease." *Cochrane Database of Systematic Reviews*, no. 3 (2020): CD003177. doi.org/10.1002/14651858.CD003177.pub5.

Altay, Ahmet, Deniz İrtem Kartal, Gökhan Sadi, Tülin Güray, and Ahmet Emre Yaprak. "Modulation of mRNA Expression and Activities of Xenobiotic Metabolizing Enzymes, CYP1A1, CYP1A2, CYP2E1, GPx and GSTP1 by the *Salicornia freitagii* Extract in HT-29 Human Colon Cancer Cells." *Archives of Biological Sciences* 69, no. 3 (2017): 439–48. doi.org/10.2298/abs160825118a.

American Heart Association. "Added Sugars." Last modified April 17, 2018. Heart.org/en/healthy-living/healthy-eating/eat-smart/sugar/added-sugars.

American Heart Association. "How Much Sugar Is Too Much?" Heart.org /en/healthy-living/healthy-eating/eat-smart/sugar/how-much-sugar -is-too-much.

American Heart Association. "Saturated Fat." Heart.org/en/healthy-living /healthy-eating/eat-smart/fats/saturated-fats.

American Heart Association. "Sodium." Last modified June 28, 2018. Heart.org/en/healthy-living/healthy-eating/eat-smart/sodium.

American Institute for Cancer Research. "Soy: Intake Does Not Increase Risk for Breast Cancer Survivors." Last modified December 30, 2019. AICR.org/cancer-prevention/food-facts/soy.

Anderson, Elizabeth, and J. Larry Durstine. "Physical Activity, Exercise, and Chronic Diseases: A Brief Review." *Sports Medicine and Health Science* 1, no. 1 (December 2019): 3–10. doi.org/10.1016/j.smhs.2019.08.006.

Ayeleso, Taiwo Betty, Khosi Ramachela, and Emmanuel Mukwevho. "A Review of Therapeutic Potentials of Sweet Potato: Pharmacological Activities and Influence of the Cultivar." *Tropical Journal of Pharmaceutical Research* 15, no. 12 (December 2016): 2751–61. doi.org/10.4314/tjpr.v15i12.31.

Azqueta, Amaya, and Andrew Collins. "Polyphenols and DNA Damage: A Mixed Blessing." *Nutrients* 8, vol. 12 (December 2016): 785. doi.org /10.3390/nu8120785.

Bae, Yong-Soo, Eui-Cheol Shin, Yoe-Sik Bae, and Willem Van Eden. "Editorial: Stress and Immunity." *Frontiers in Immunology* 10 (February 2019): 245. doi.org/10.3389/fimmu.2019.00245.

Bousseau, Simon, Luisa Vergori, Raffaella Soleti, Guy Lenaers, M. Carmen Martinez, and Ramaroson Andriantsitohaina. "Glycosylation as New Pharmacological Strategies for Diseases Associated with Excessive Angiogenesis." *Pharmacology & Therapeutics* 191 (November 2018): 92–122. doi.org/10.1016/j.pharmthera.2018.06.003.

Busnelli, Marco, Stefano Manzini, Cesare R. Sirtori, Giulia Chiesa, and Cinzia Parolini. "Effects of Vegetable Proteins on Hypercholesterolemia and Gut Microbiota Modulation." *Nutrients* 10, no. 9 (September 2018): 1249. doi.org/10.3390/nu10091249.

Cano-Lamadrid, M., F. C. Marhuenda-Egea, F. Hernández, E. C. Rosas-Burgos, A. Burgos-Hernández, and A. A. Carbonell-Barrachina. "Biological Activity of Conventional and Organic Pomegranate Juices: Antioxidant and Antimutagenic Potential." *Plant Foods for Human Nutrition* 71 (December 2016): 375–80. doi.org/10.1007/s11130-016-0569-y.

Cao, Yanan, Liang Zou, Wei Li, Yu Song, Gang Zhao, and Yichen Hu. "Dietary Quinoa (*Chenopodium quinoa* Willd.) Polysaccharides Ameliorate High-Fat Diet-Induced Hyperlipidemia and Modulate Gut Microbiota." *International Journal of Biological Macromolecules* 163 (November 2020): 55–65. doi.org/10.1016/j.ijbiomac.2020.06.241.

Centers for Disease Control and Prevention. "What Are the Risk Factors for Lung Cancer?" Last modified September 22, 2020. CDC.gov/cancer/lung/basic_info/risk_factors.htm.

Challa, Hima J., Muhammad Atif Ameer, and Kalyan R. Uppaluri. *DASH Diet to Stop Hypertension*. Treasure Island, FL: StatPearls Publishing, 2018.

Chen, Qing-Fu, Xiao-Yan Huang, Hong-You Li, Li-Juan Yang, and Ya-Song Cui. "Recent Progress in Perennial Buckwheat Development." *Sustainability* 10, no. 2 (February 2018): 536. doi.org/10.3390/su10020536.

Clark, Michael A., Marco Springmann, Jason Hill, and David Tilman. "Multiple Health and Environmental Impacts of Foods." *Proceedings of the National Academy of Sciences of the United States of America* 116, no. 46 (November 2019): 23357–62. doi.org/10.1073/pnas.1906908116.

Davis, Cindy D. "The Gut Microbiome and Its Role in Obesity." *Nutrition Today* 51, no. 4 (July/August 2016): 167–74. doi.org/10.1097/NT.0000000000000167.

De Gaetano, G., S. Costanzo, A. Di Castelnuovo, L. Badimon, D. Bejko, A. Alkerwi, G. Chiva-Blanch, et al. "Effects of Moderate Beer Consumption on Health and Disease: A Consensus Document." *Nutrition, Metabolism & Cardiovascular Diseases* 26, no. 6 (June 2016): 443–67. doi.org/10.1016/j.numecd.2016.03.007.

Delaware Sea Grant. "Seafood Health Facts: Making Smart Choices." SeafoodHealthFacts.org/seafood-nutrition/healthcare-professionals/omega-3-content-frequently-consumed-seafood-products.

Dobner, J., and S. Kaser. "Body Mass Index and the Risk of Infection—From Underweight to Obesity." *Clinical Microbiology and Infection* 24, no. 1 (January 2018): 24–28. doi.org/10.1016/j.cmi.2017.02.013.

Fang, Mingzhu, Dapeng Chen, and Chung S. Yang. "Dietary Polyphenols May Affect DNA Methylation." *Journal of Nutrition* 137, no. 1 (January 2007): 223S–28S. doi.org/10.1093/jn/137.1.223S.

Fatima, Tabasum, Beenish, Bazila Naseer, Gousia Gani, Tahiya Qadri, and Tashooq Ah Bhat. "Antioxidant Potential and Health Benefits of Cumin." *Journal of Medicinal Plants Studies* 6, no. 2 (2018): 232–36. PlantsJournal .com/archives/2018/vol6issue2/PartD/6-2-28-858.pdf.

Ferrer, Manuel, Celia Méndez-García, David Rojo, Coral Barbas, and Andrés Moya. "Antibiotic Use and Microbiome Function." *Biochemical Pharmacology* 134 (June 2017): 114–26. doi.org/10.1016/j.bcp.2016.09.007.

Fiorenza, M., L. Gliemann, N. Brandt, and J. Bangsbo. "Hormetic Modula-tion of Angiogenic Factors by Exercise-Induced Mechanical and Metabolic Stress in Human Skeletal Muscle." *American Journal of Physiology—Heart and Circulatory Physiology* 319, no. 4 (October 2020): H824–34. doi.org/10.1152/ajpheart.00432.2020.

Fujiki, Hirota, Tatsuro Watanabe, Eisaburo Sueoka, Anchalee Rawangkan, and Masami Suganuma. "Cancer Prevention with Green Tea and Its Principal Constituent, EGCG: From Early Investigations to Current Focus on Human Cancer Stem Cells." *Molecules and Cells* 41, no. 2 (2018): 73–82. doi.org/10.14348/molcells.2018.2227.

Ghiţu, Alexandra, Anja Schwiebs, Heinfried H. Radeke, Stefana Avram, Istvan Zupko, Andrea Bor, Ioana Zinuca Pavel, et al. "A Comprehensive Assessment of Apigenin as an Antiproliferative, Proapoptotic, Antiangiogenic and Immunomodulatory Phytocompound." *Nutrients* 11, no. 4 (April 2019): 858. doi.org/10.3390/nu11040858.

Ghosh, Shampa, Jitendra Kumar Sinha, and Manchala Raghunath. "Epigenomic Maintenance through Dietary Intervention Can Facilitate DNA Repair Process to Slow Down the Progress of Premature Aging." *IUBMB Life* 68, no. 9 (September 2016): 717–21. doi.org/10.1002/iub.1532.

Gunter, Marc J., Neil Murphy, Amanda J. Cross, Laure Dossus, Laureen Dartois, Guy Fagherazzi, Rudolf Kaaks, et al. "Coffee Drinking and Mortality in 10 European Countries: A Multinational Cohort Study." *Annals of Internal Medicine* 167, no. 4 (August 2017): 236–47. doi.org/10.7326/M16-2945.

Habib, Mohammad Asadul, Kawsar Hossen, and Md. Al Amin. "Anti-Carcinogenic Effect of Lemon & Lemon Products in Cancer Therapy: A Summary of the Evidence." *International Journal of Trend in Scientific Research and Development* 3, no. 6 (October 2019): 1261–66. doi.org/10.13140/RG.2.2.27108.12168.

Händel, Mina Nicole, Isabel Cardoso, Katrine Marie Rasmussen, Jeanett Friis Rohde, Ramune Jacobsen, Sabrina Mai Nielsen, Robin Christensen, and Berit Lilienthal Heitmann. "Processed Meat Intake and Chronic Disease Morbidity and Mortality: An Overview of Systematic Reviews and Meta-Analyses." *PLOS One* 14, no. 10 (October 2019): e0223883. doi.org/10.1371/journal.pone.0223883.

Haspel, Jeffrey A., Ron Anafi, Marishka K. Brown, Nicolas Cermakian, Christopher Depner, Paula Desplats, Andrew E. Gelman, et al. "Perfect Timing: Circadian Rhythms, Sleep, and Immunity—An NIH Workshop Summary." *Journal of Clinical Investigation Insight* 5, no. 1 (January 2020): e131487. doi.org/10.1172/jci.insight.131487.

Heiss, Christian, Nicolas Amabile, Andrew C. Lee, Wendy May Real, Suzaynn F. Schick, David Lao, Maelene L. Wong, et al. "Brief Secondhand Smoke Exposure Depresses Endothelial Progenitor Cells Activity and Endothelial Function: Sustained Vascular Injury and Blunted Nitric Oxide Production." *Journal of the American College of Cardiology* 51, no. 18 (May 2008): 1760–71. doi.org/10.1016/j.jacc.2008.01.040.

Henning, Susanne M., Jieping Yang, Paul Shao, Ru-Po Lee, Jianjun Huang, Austin Ly, Mark Hsu, et al. "Health Benefit of Vegetable/Fruit Juice-Based Diet: Role of Microbiome." *Scientific Reports* 7 (May 2017): 2167. doi.org/10.1038/s41598-017-02200-6.

Hess, Julie M., Satya S. Jonnalagadda, and Joanne L. Slavin. "What Is a Snack, Why Do We Snack, and How Can We Choose Better Snacks? A Review of the Definitions of Snacking, Motivations to Snack, Contributions to Dietary Intake, and Recommendations for Improvement." *Advances in Nutrition* 7, no. 3 (May 2016): 466–75. doi.org/10.3945/an.115.009571.

Hooshmand-Moghadam, Babak, Mozhgan Eskandari, Fateme Golestani, Saeed Rezae, Nahid Mahmoudi, and Abbas Ali Gaeini. "The Effect of 12-Week Resistance Exercise Training on Serum Levels of Cellular Aging Process Parameters in Elderly Men." *Experimental Gerontology* 141 (November 2020): 111090. doi.org/10.1016/j.exger.2020.111090.

Jenkins, David J. A., Sonia Blanco Mejia, Laura Chiavaroli, Effie Viguiliouk, Siying S. Li, Cyril W. C. Kendall, Vladmir Vuksan, and John L. Sievenpiper. "Cumulative Meta-Analysis of the Soy Effect over Time." *Journal of the American Heart Association* 8, no. 13 (July 2019): e012458. doi.org/10.1161/JAHA.119.012458.

Joyce, Susan A., Alison Kamil, Lisa Fleige, and Cormac G. M. Gahan. "The Cholesterol-Lowering Effect of Oats and Oat Beta Glucan: Modes of Action and Potential Role of Bile Acids and the Microbiome." *Frontiers in Nutrition* 6 (November 2019): 171. doi.org/10.3389/fnut.2019.00171.

Juskowiak, Bogna, Anna Bogacz, Marlena Wolek, Adam Kamiński, Izabela Uzar, Agnieszka Seremak-Mrozikiewicz, and Bogusław Czerny. "Expression Profiling of Genes Modulated by Rosmarinic Acid (RA) in MCF-7 Breast Cancer Cells." *Ginekologia Polska* 89, no. 10 (2018): 541–45. doi.org/10.5603/GP.a2018.0092.

Kapadiya Dhartiben, B., and K. D. Aparnathi. "Chemistry and Use of Artificial Intense Sweeteners." *International Journal of Current Microbiology and Applied Sciences* 6, no. 6 (2017): 1283–96. doi.org/10.20546/ijcmas.2017.606.151.

Khan, Israr, Naeem Ullah, Lajia Zha, Yanrui Bai, Ashiq Khan, Tang Zhao, Tuanjie Che, and Chunjiang Zhang. "Alteration of Gut Microbiota in Inflammatory Bowel Disease (IBD): Cause or Consequence? IBD Treatment Targeting the Gut Microbiome." *Pathogens* 8, no. 3 (September 2019): 126. doi.org/10.3390/pathogens8030126.

Kobrynski, Lisa, Rachel Waltenburg Powell, and Scott Bowen. "Prevalence and Morbidity of Primary Immunodeficiency Diseases, United States 2001–2007." *Journal of Clinical Immunology* 34 (November 2014): 954–61. doi.org/10.1007/s10875-014-0102-8.

Kreft, Marko. "Buckwheat Phenolic Metabolites in Health and Disease." *Nutrition Research Reviews* 29, no. 1 (June 2016): 30–39. doi.org/10.1017/S0954422415000190.

Lange, Klaus W., and Yukiko Nakamura. "Food Bioactives, Micronutrients, Immune Function and COVID-19." *Journal of Food Bioactives* 10 (June 2020): 1–8. doi.org/10.31665/JFB.2020.10222.

Lerner, Aaron, Patricia Jeremias, and Torsten Matthias. "The World Incidence and Prevalence of Autoimmune Diseases Is Increasing." *International Journal of Celiac Disease* 3, no. 4 (2015): 151–55. doi.org/10.12691/ijcd-3-4-8.

Levine, Morgan E., Ake T. Lu, Austin Quach, Brian H. Chen, Themistocles L. Assimes, Stefania Bandinelli, Lifang Hou, et al. "An Epigenetic Biomarker of Aging for Lifespan and Healthspan." *Aging* 10, no. 4 (April 2018): 573–91. doi.org/10.18632/aging.101414.

Lewis, Kayla A., and Trygve O. Tollefsbol. "Regulation of the Telomerase Reverse Transcriptase Subunit through Epigenetic Mechanisms." *Frontiers in Genetics* 7 (May 2016): 83. doi.org/10.3389/fgene.2016.00083.

Li, Linshan, Ronald B. Pegg, Ronald R. Eitenmiller, Ji-Yeon Chun, and Adrian L. Kerrihard. "Selected Nutrient Analyses of Fresh, Fresh-Stored, and Frozen Fruits and Vegetables." *Journal of Food Composition and Analysis* 59 (June 2017): 8–17. doi.org/10.1016/j.jfca.2017.02.002.

Li, William W. *Eat to Beat Disease: The New Science of How Your Body Can Heal Itself*. New York: Grand Central Publishing, 2019.

Luo, Haitao, Bing-Hua Jiang, Sarah M. King, and Yi Charlie Chen. "Inhibition of Cell Growth and VEGF Expression in Ovarian Cancer Cells by Flavonoids." *Nutrition and Cancer* 60, no. 6 (2008): 800–809. doi.org/10.1080/01635580802100851.

Mahassni, Sawsan Hassan, and Oroob Abid Bukhari. "Beneficial Effects of an Aqueous Ginger Extract on the Immune System Cells and Antibodies, Hematology, and Thyroid Hormones in Male Smokers and Non-Smokers." *Journal of Nutrition & Intermediary Metabolism* 15 (March 2019): 10–17. doi.org/10.1016/j.jnim.2018.10.001.

Mahmood, Ahmed M., and Hayder B. Sahib. "Anti-Angiogenic Activity of *Cuminum cyminum* Seeds Extract: *In Vivo* Study." *Kerbala Journal of Pharmaceutical Sciences* 13 (2017): 1–9. IASJ.net/iasj/download /387965e93204bc95.

Manchali, Shivapriya, Kotamballi N. Chidambara Murthy, and Bhimanagouda S. Patil. "Crucial Facts about Health Benefits of Popular Cruciferous Vegetables." *Journal of Functional Foods* 4, no. 1 (January 2012): 94–106. doi.org/10.1016/j.jff.2011.08.004.

Marco, Maria L., Dustin Heeney, Sylvie Binda, Christopher J. Cifelli, Paul D. Cotter, Benoit Foligné, Michael Gänzle et al. "Health Benefits of Fermented Foods: Microbiota and Beyond." *Current Opinion in Biotechnology* 44 (April 2017): 94–102. doi.org/10.1016/j.copbio.2016.11.010.

Martínez-Villaluenga, Cristina, and Elena Peñas. "Health Benefits of Oat: Current Evidence and Molecular Mechanisms." *Current Opinion in Food Science* 14 (April 2017): 26–31. doi.org/10.1016/j.cofs.2017.01.004.

Mason, Ashley E., Jonathan M. Adler, Eli Puterman, Ava Lakmazaheri, Matthew Brucker, Kirstin Aschbacher, and Elissa S. Epel. "Stress Resilience: Narrative Identity May Buffer the Longitudinal Effects of Chronic Caregiving Stress on Mental Health and Telomere Shortening." *Brain, Behavior, and Immunity* 77 (March 2019): 101–9. doi.org/10.1016/j .bbi.2018.12.010.

McClain, Justin A., Dayna M. Hayes, Stephanie A. Morris, and Kimberly Nixon. "Adolescent Binge Alcohol Exposure Alters Hippocampal Progenitor Cell Proliferation in Rats: Effects on Cell Cycle Kinetics." *Journal of Comparative Neurology* 519, no. 13 (September 2011): 2697–710. doi.org /10.1002/cne.22647.

Melina, Vesanto, Winston Craig, and Susan Levin. "Position of the Academy of Nutrition and Dietetics: Vegetarian Diets." *Journal of the Academy of Nutrition and Dietetics* 116, no. 12 (December 2016): 1970–80. doi.org /10.1016/j.jand.2016.09.025.

Mellor, Duane D., Bishoy Hanna-Khalil, and Raymond Carson. "A Review of the Potential Health Benefits of Low Alcohol and Alcohol-Free Beer: Effects of Ingredients and Craft Brewing Processes on Potentially Bioactive

Metabolites." *Beverages* 6, no. 2 (June 2020): 25. doi.org/10.3390
/beverages6020025.

Milani, Christian, Sabrina Duranti, Stefania Napoli, Giulia Alessandri,
Leonardo Mancabelli, Rosaria Anzalone, Giulia Longhi, et al. "Colonization
of the Human Gut by Bovine Bacteria Present in Parmesan Cheese." *Nature
Communications* 10 (2019): 1286. doi.org/10.1038/s41467-019-09303-w.

Milo, Ron, and Rob Phillips. "Rates and Durations." In *Cell Biology by
the Numbers*, 278–82. New York: Garland Science, Taylor & Francis
Group, 2015.

Mitra, Sumonto, and Shashi Khandelwal. "Health Benefits of Tea: Beneficial
Effects of Tea on Human Health." In *Exploring the Nutrition and Health
Benefits of Functional Foods*, ed. Hossain Uddin Shekhar, Zakir Hossain
Howlader, and Yearul Kabir, 99–116. Hershey, PA: IGI Global, 2017.

Mohajeri, M. Hasan, Robert J. M. Brummer, Robert A. Rastall, Rinse K.
Weersma, Hermie J. M. Harmsen, Marijke Faas, and Manfred Eggersdorfer.
"The Role of the Microbiome for Human Health: From Basic Science to Clinical Applications." *European Journal of Nutrition* 57 (May 2018): 1–14. doi.org
/10.1007/s00394-018-1703-4.

Monterey Bay Aquarium Seafood Watch. "Helping People Make Better
Choices for a Healthy Ocean." SeafoodWatch.org/about-us.

Nash, Victoria, C. Senaka Ranadheera, Ekavi N. Georgousopoulou, Duane D.
Mellor, Demosthenes B. Panagiotakos, Andrew J. McKune, Jane Kellett,
and Nenad Naumovski. "The Effects of Grape and Red Wine Polyphenols
on Gut Microbiota—A Systematic Review." *Food Research International* 113
(November 2018): 277–87. doi.org/10.1016/j.foodres.2018.07.019.

National Cancer Institute. "Chemicals in Meat Cooked at High
Temperatures and Cancer Risk." Last modified July 11, 2017. cancer.gov
/about-cancer/causes-prevention/risk/diet/cooked-meats-fact-sheet.

National Heart, Lung, and Blood Institute. "Your Guide to Healthy Sleep."
Last modified August 2011. NHLBI.NIH.gov/files/docs/public/sleep
/healthy_sleep.pdf.

National Institute of Environmental Health Sciences. "Autoimmune Diseases." Last modified May 6, 2020. NIEHS.NIH.gov/health/topics /conditions/autoimmune/index.cfm.

Okonkwo, Uzoagu A., and Luisa A. DiPietro. "Diabetes and Wound Angiogenesis." *International Journal of Molecular Sciences* 18, no. 7 (July 2017): 1419. doi.org/10.3390/ijms18071419.

Peirce, Jason M., and Karina Alviña. "The Role of Inflammation and the Gut Microbiome in Depression and Anxiety." *Journal of Neuroscience Research* 97, no. 10 (October 2019): 1223–41. doi.org/10.1002/jnr.24476.

Penn, J. S., A. Madan, R. B. Caldwell, M. Bartoli, R. W. Caldwell, and M. E. Hartnett. "Vascular Endothelial Growth Factor in Eye Disease." *Progress in Retinal and Eye Research* 27, no. 4 (July 2008): 331–71. doi.org/10.1016 /j.preteyeres.2008.05.001.

Pérez-Cano, Francisco J., Malen Massot-Cladera, Àngels Franch, Cristina Castellote, and Margarida Castell. "The Effects of Cocoa on the Immune System." *Frontiers in Pharmacology* 4 (June 2013): 71. doi.org /10.3389/fphar.2013.00071.

Poswal, Fatima S., Grace Russell, Marion Mackonochie, Euan MacLennan, Emmanuel C. Adukwu, and Vivien Rolfe. "Herbal Teas and Their Health Benefits: A Scoping Review." *Plant Foods for Human Nutrition* 74 (September 2019): 266–76. doi.org/10.1007/s11130-019-00750-w.

Potz, Brittany A., Anshul B. Parulkar, Ruhul M. Abid, Neel R. Sodha, and Frank W. Sellke. "Novel Molecular Targets for Coronary Angiogenesis and Ischemic Heart Disease." *Coronary Artery Disease* 28, no. 7 (November 2017): 605–13. doi.org/10.1097/MCA.0000000000000516.

Prasad, Kedar N., Meixia Wu, and Stephen C. Bondy. "Telomere Shortening during Aging: Attenuation by Antioxidants and Anti-Inflammatory Agents." *Mechanisms of Ageing and Development* 164 (June 2017): 61–66. doi.org /10.1016/j.mad.2017.04.004.

Quesada-Molina, Mar, Araceli Muñoz-Garach, Francisco J. Tinahones, and Isabel Moreno-Indias. "A New Perspective on the Health Benefits of Moderate Beer Consumption: Involvement of the Gut Microbiota." *Metabolites* 9, no. 11 (November 2019): 272. doi.org/10.3390 /metabo9110272.

Saeed, Brhaish Ali, Vuanghao Lim, Nor Adlin Yusof, Kang Zi Khor, Heshu Sulaiman Rahman, and Nozlena Abdul Samad. "Antiangiogenic Properties of Nanoparticles: A Systematic Review." *International Journal of Nanomedicine* 14 (2019): 5135–46. doi.org/10.2147/ijn.s199974.

Sakai, Chiemi, Mari Ishida, Hideo Ohba, Hiromitsu Yamashita, Hitomi Uchida, Masao Yoshizumi, and Takafumi Ishida. "Fish Oil Omega-3 Polyunsaturated Fatty Acids Attenuate Oxidative Stress-Induced DNA Damage in Vascular Endothelial Cells." *PLOS One* 12, no. 11 (November 2017): e0187934. doi.org/10.1371/journal.pone.0187934.

Sánchez-Sánchez, María Luz, Alicia García-Vigara, Juan José Hidalgo-Mora, Miguel-Ángel García-Pérez, Juan Tarín, and Antonio Cano. "Mediterranean Diet and Health: A Systematic Review of Epidemiological Studies and Intervention Trials." *Maturitas* 136 (June 2020): 25–37. doi.org/10.1016/j .maturitas.2020.03.008.

Savoye, Isabelle, Catherine M. Olsen, David C. Whiteman, Anne Bijon, Lucien Wald, Laureen Dartois, Françoise Clavel-Chapelon, Marie-Christine Boutron-Ruault, and Marina Kvaskoff. "Patterns of Ultraviolet Radiation Exposure and Skin Cancer Risk: The E3N-SunExp Study." *Journal of Epidemiology* 28, no. 1 (2018): 27–33. doi.org/10.2188/jea.JE20160166.

Schwingshackl, Lukas, Anna Chaimani, Angela Bechthold, Khalid Iqbal, Marta Stelmach-Mardas, Georg Hoffmann, Carolina Schwedhelm, Sabrina Schlesinger, and Heiner Boeing. "Food Groups and Risk of Chronic Disease: A Protocol for a Systematic Review and Network Meta-Analysis of Cohort Studies." *Systematic Reviews* 5 (2016): 125. doi.org/10.1186 /s13643-016-0302-9.

Seattle Cancer Care Alliance. "Blood and Marrow Transplant." SeattleCCA .org/treatments/bone-marrow-transplant.

Sender, Ron, Shai Fuchs, and Ron Milo. "Revised Estimates for the Number of Human and Bacteria Cells in the Body." *PLOS Biology* 14, no. 8 (August 2016): e1002533. doi.org/10.1371/journal.pbio.1002533.

Shammas, Masood A. "Telomeres, Lifestyle, Cancer, and Aging." *Current Opinion in Clinical Nutrition and Metabolic Care* 14, no. 1 (January 2011): 28–34. doi.org/10.1097/MCO.0b013e32834121b1.

Simon, Stacy. "How Your Diet May Affect Your Risk of Breast Cancer." American Cancer Society, October 1, 2018. Cancer.org/latest-news /how-your-diet-may-affect-your-risk-of-breast-cancer.html.

Simpson, Richard J., John P. Campbell, Maree Gleeson, Karsten Krüger, David C. Nieman, David B. Pyne, James E. Turner, and Neil P. Walsh. "Can Exercise Affect Immune Function to Increase Susceptibility to Infection?" *Exercise Immunology Review* 26 (2020): 8–22. EIR-ISEI.de/2020/eir -2020-008-article.pdf.

Smith, Robert P., Cole Easson, Sarah M. Lyle, Ritishka Kapoor, Chase P. Donnelly, Eileen J. Davidson, Esha Parikh, Jose V. Lopez, and Jaime L. Tartar. "Gut Microbiome Diversity Is Associated with Sleep Physiology in Humans." *PLOS One* 14, no. 10 (October 2019): e0222394. doi.org/10.1371 /journal.pone.0222394.

Snopek, Lukas, Jiri Mlcek, Lenka Sochorova, Mojmir Baron, Irena Hlavacova, Tunde Jurikova, Rene Kizek, Eva Sedlackova, and Jiri Sochor. "Contribution of Red Wine Consumption to Human Health Protection." *Molecules* 23, no. 7 (July 2018): 1684. doi.org/10.3390/molecules23071684.

Stenholm, Sari, Jenny Head, Mika Kivimäki, Linda L. Magnusson Hanson, Jaana Pentti, Naja H. Rod, Alice J. Clark, Tuula Oksanen, Hugo Westerlund, and Jussi Vahtera. "Sleep Duration and Sleep Disturbances as Predictors of Healthy and Chronic Disease-Free Life Expectancy between Ages 50 and 75: A Pooled Analysis of Three Cohorts." *Journals of Gerontology: Series A* 74, no. 2 (February 2019): 204–10. doi.org/10.1093/gerona/gly016.

Tajik, Narges, Mahboubeh Tajik, Isabelle Mack, and Paul Enck. "The Potential Effects of Chlorogenic Acid, the Main Phenolic Components in Coffee, on Health: A Comprehensive Review of the Literature." *European Journal of Nutrition* 56 (October 2017): 2215–44. doi.org/10.1007/s00394-017-1379-1.

Thompson, Sharon V., Melisa A. Bailey, Andrew M. Taylor, Jennifer L. Kaczmarek, Annemarie R. Mysonhimer, Caitlyn G. Edwards, Ginger E. Reeser, Nicholas A. Burd, Naiman A. Khan, and Hannah D. Holscher. "Avocado Consumption Alters Gastrointestinal Bacteria Abundance and Microbial Metabolite Concentrations among Adults with Overweight or Obesity: A Randomized Controlled Trial." *Journal of Nutrition* (2020): nxaa219. doi.org/10.1093/jn/nxaa219.

Toda, Masaaki, Toshiaki Totoki, Chizu Nakamura, Taro Yasuma, Corina N. D'Alessandro-Gabazza, Rumi Mifuji-Moroka, Kota Nishihama, et al. "Low Dose of Alcohol Attenuates Pro-Atherosclerotic Activity of Thrombin." *Atherosclerosis* 265 (October 2017): 215–24. doi.org/10.1016/j.atherosclerosis.2017.09.005.

Torre, Elisa, Giorgio Iviglia, Clara Cassinelli, Marco Morra, and Nazario Russo. "Polyphenols from Grape Pomace Induce Osteogenic Differentiation in Mesenchymal Stem Cells." *International Journal of Molecular Medicine* 45, no. 6 (June 2020): 1721–34. doi.org/10.3892/ijmm.2020.4556.

Turgeon, Julie, Sylvie Dussault, Fritz Maingrette, Jessika Groleau, Paola Haddad, Gemma Perez, and Alain Rivard. "Fish Oil–Enriched Diet Protects against Ischemia by Improving Angiogenesis, Endothelial Progenitor Cell Function and Postnatal Neovascularization." *Atherosclerosis* 229, no. 2 (August 2013): 295–303. doi.org/10.1016/j.atherosclerosis.2013.05.020.

US Department of Health and Human Services. *Physical Activity Guidelines for Americans, 2nd edition.* Washington, DC: US Department of Health and Human Services, 2018. Health.gov/sites/default/files/2019-09/Physical_Activity_Guidelines_2nd_edition.pdf.

Usta, Coskun, Semir Ozdemir, Michele Schiariti, and Paolo Emilio Puddu. "The Pharmacological Use of Ellagic Acid-Rich Pomegranate Fruit." *International Journal of Food Sciences and Nutrition* 64, no. 7 (November 2013): 907–13. doi.org/10.3109/09637486.2013.798268.

Valitutti, Francesco, Salvatore Cucchiara, and Alessio Fasano. "Celiac Disease and the Microbiome." *Nutrients* 11, no. 10 (October 2019): 2403. doi.org/10.3390/nu11102403.

Vigsnæs, Louise Kristine, Jesper Holck, Anne S. Meyer, and Tine Rask Licht. "*In Vitro* Fermentation of Sugar Beet Arabino-Oligosaccharides by Fecal Microbiota Obtained from Patients with Ulcerative Colitis to Selectively Stimulate the Growth of *Bifidobacterium* spp. and *Lactobacillus* spp." *Applied and Environmental Microbiology* 77, no. 23 (December 2011): 8336–44. doi.org/10.1128/AEM.05895-11.

Volokh, Olesya, Natalia Klimenko, Yulia Berezhnaya, Alexander Tyakht, Polina Nesterova, Anna Popenko, and Dmitry Alexeev. "Human Gut Microbiome Response Induced by Fermented Dairy Product Intake in Healthy Volunteers." *Nutrients* 11, no. 3 (March 2019): 547. doi.org/10.3390/nu11030547.

Wang, Dong, LeeAnn K. Li, Tiffany Dai, Aijun Wang, and Song Li. "Adult Stem Cells in Vascular Remodeling." *Theranostics* 8, no. 3 (2018): 815–29. doi.org/10.7150/thno.19577.

Watanabe, Shaw, and Mari Uehara. "Health Effects and Safety of Soy and Isoflavones." In *The Role of Functional Food Security in Global Health,* ed. Ram B. Singh, Ronald Ross Watson, and Toru Takahashi, 379–94. San Diego: Academic Press, 2019. doi.org/10.1016/B978-0-12-813148-0.00022-0.

Weng, Mao-wen, Hyun-Wook Lee, Sung-Hyun Park, Yu Hu, Hsing-Tsui Wang, Lung-Chi Chen, William N. Rom, et al. "Aldehydes Are the Predominant Forces Inducing DNA Damage and Inhibiting DNA Repair in Tobacco Smoke Carcinogenesis." *Proceedings of the National Academy of Sciences of the United States of America* 115, no. 27 (July 2018): E6152–61. doi.org/10.1073/pnas.1804869115.

Wojcicki, Janet M., Rosalinda Medrano, Jue Lin, and Elissa Epel. "Increased Cellular Aging by 3 Years of Age in Latino, Preschool Children Who Consume More Sugar-Sweetened Beverages: A Pilot Study." *Childhood Obesity* 14, no. 3 (April 2018): 149–57. doi.org/10.1089/chi.2017.0159.

Xiang, Huan, Dongxiao Sun-Waterhouse, Geoffrey I. N. Waterhouse, Chun Cui, and Zheng Ruan. "Fermentation-Enabled Wellness Foods: A Fresh Perspective." *Food Science and Human Wellness* 8, no. 3 (September 2019): 203–43. doi.org/10.1016/j.fshw.2019.08.003.

Yamagata, Kazuo, Yuri Izawa, Daiki Onodera, and Motoki Tagami. "Chlorogenic Acid Regulates Apoptosis and Stem Cell Marker-Related Gene Expression in A549 Human Lung Cancer Cells." *Molecular and Cellular Biochemistry* 441 (2018): 9–19. doi.org/10.1007/s11010-017-3171-1.

Yang, Jiali, Lingrong Wen, Yueming Jiang, and Bao Yang. "Natural Estrogen Receptor Modulators and Their Heterologous Biosynthesis." *Trends in Endocrinology & Metabolism* 30, no. 1 (January 2019): 66–76. doi.org/10.1016/j.tem.2018.11.002.

Yang, Ji Won, and Il Sook Choi. "Comparison of the Phenolic Composition and Antioxidant Activity of Korean Black Raspberry, Bokbunja (*Rubus coreanus* Miquel) with Those of Six Other Berries." *CyTA Journal of Food* 15, no. 1 (2017): 110–17. doi.org/10.1080/19476337.2016.1219390.

Zaheer, Khalid, and M. Humayoun Akhtar. "An Updated Review of Dietary Isoflavones: Nutrition, Processing, Bioavailability and Impacts on Human Health." *Critical Reviews in Food Science and Nutrition* 57, no. 6 (2017): 1280–93. doi.org/10.1080/10408398.2014.989958.

Zamora-Ros, Raul, Dinesh K. Barupal, Joseph A. Rothwell, Mazda Jenab, Veronika Fedirko, Isabelle Romieu, Krasimira Aleksandrova, et al. "Dietary Flavonoid Intake and Colorectal Cancer Risk in the European Prospective Investigation into Cancer and Nutrition (EPIC) Cohort." *International Journal of Cancer* 140, no. 8 (April 2017): 1836–44. doi.org/10.1002/ijc.30582.

Zhang, Cheng, Ning Wang, Hor-Yue Tan, Wei Guo, Sha Li, and Yibin Feng. "Targeting VEGF/VEGFRs Pathway in the Antiangiogenic Treatment of Human Cancers by Traditional Chinese Medicine." *Integrative Cancer Therapies* 17, no. 3 (2018): 582–601. doi.org/10.1177/1534735418775828.

Zheng, Jinshui, Xin Zhao, Xiaoxi B. Lin, and Michael Gänzle. "Comparative Genomics *Lactobacillus reuteri* from Sourdough Reveals Adaptation of an Intestinal Symbiont to Food Fermentations." *Scientific Reports* 5 (December 2015): 18234. doi.org/10.1038/srep18234.

INDEX

ACKNOWLEDGMENTS

So many wonderful supporters helped make this book possible. Trevor, I couldn't do this without you. Thank you for taste-testing and for validating that a couple of the recipes in this book are your "favorites I've ever made." To my Mom, Cheryle, you tested and tested even during a move, and I greatly appreciate your culinary expertise, as always. My Dad, Greg's, taste-testing validated the recipes that ultimately make up this book today. Thank you for your constant support and encouragement.

I want to thank the International Ladies Cari, Jen, Stefanie, Kendra, and Marissa; HH's Julia, Aileen, Laura; Jessica and Sharon; Lacey, Sara M, Rachel D, Julie, and Erica. Your testing and honest feedback made all of this possible. Your energy lives in this book! To my interns Taryn, Mia, and Taylor: thank you, and I appreciate you so much. You're going to be amazing dietitians someday soon, and I'm honored that you were there to be a part of this project.

To cousin Kylie, whom we lost while I was working on this project, your light will be missed. Your passion for health and fitness lives on in so many others.

Thank you to my wonderful agent, Marilyn, at Allen Literary Agency and to my team at Callisto Media for all their hard work and collaboration on this project.

ABOUT THE AUTHOR

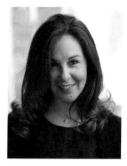

Ginger Hultin, MS, RDN, is a registered dietitian nutritionist and owner of the Seattle-based virtual nutrition practices Champagne Nutrition®, where she educates based on the balance of including foods her clients love within a healthy lifestyle that helps them meet their goals, and Seattle Cancer Nutritionist, where she serves as an integrative oncology nutrition specialist. She runs the food blog at Champagne Nutrition® and is a national expert voice in the media. Her many interviews on nutrition and health have appeared in the *Washington Post*, Food Network, *HuffPost*, CNN, *Reader's Digest*, *Wine Spectator*, and many others. She speaks regularly about nutrition and health to large audiences around the world, including in Chicago, Illinois; Austin, Texas; Los Angeles, California; Beirut, Lebanon; Amman, Jordan; and Kuwait City, Kuwait.

Ginger completed her undergraduate degree in English literature at the University of Washington and earned a master's degree in nutrition from Bastyr University. A Pacific Northwest native, she resides in Seattle, where she serves as president of the board of her local dietetic association affiliate, the Greater Seattle Dietetic Association, and is an advisory board member of Team Survivor Northwest. When she's not focused on her nutrition work and volunteer activities, you can find her on her Peloton bike or taking care of her adopted senior cat.

Ginger believes in the healing power of food and has seen dietary changes alter the course of many clients' health. Her years in clinical practice, specializing in nutrigenomics, oncology nutrition, autoimmune conditions, and cardiac health, have led to a passion around educating clients to use nutrition as part of their care plan. Follow her on Instagram, Pinterest, and Facebook @ChampagneNutrition, on Twitter @GingerHultinRD, and on her blog at ChampagneNutrition.com.

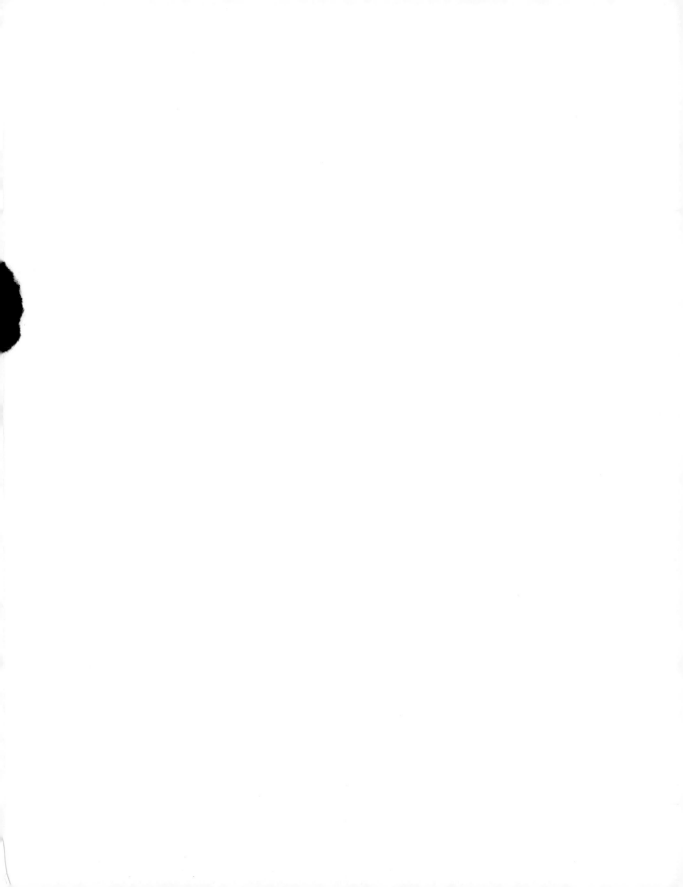